Where There's Life,
There's Life

ALSO BY DAVID M. FELDMAN

*Birth Control in Jewish Law: Marital Relations,
Contraception, and Abortion as Set Forth in the Classic
Texts of Jewish Law*

*Health and Medicine in the Jewish Tradition:
L'hayyim—To Life*

Readers can contact the author via e-mail at
RabbiFeldman@YasharBooks.com

Where There's Life, There's Life

David M. Feldman

Yashar Books ♦ 2006
Brooklyn, NY

Where There's, Life There's Life

Second printing, April 2006

Library of Congress Cataloging-in-Publication Data

Feldman, David M. (David Michael)
  Where There's Life, There's Life / by David M. Feldman
  p. cm.
  1. Medicine—Religious aspects—Judaism. 2. Medical ethics. 3. Ethics, Jewish. 4. Medical laws and legislation (Jewish law).
  I. Feldman, David M.
ISBN 1-933143-11-8

For information and catalog write to Yashar Books Inc., 1548 E. 33rd Street, Brooklyn, NY 11234, or visit our website: www.YasharBooks.com

TABLE OF CONTENTS

"This is a time for sanctification of life, kiddush ha-chayyim, not for the holiness of death, kiddush ha-Shem. Previously, the oppressor demanded our soul, and we answered with martyrdom. Now, our body is demanded, and we must answer by defending it, by preserving life."

—Rabbi Isaac Nissenbaum, addressing his followers on the night before the Warsaw Ghetto uprising, April 1943

PREFACE

The reasons and need for this book are manifold. Chapter One begins with an incident that launched the book's conception and composition, but the canvas of its response is much broader. The issues are eternal and current, and the need to address them is both urgent and constant. So, as with previous efforts—*Birth Control in Jewish Law* and *Health and Medicine in the Jewish Tradition*—I offer this volume with pride and enthusiasm. In the many sessions of public lectures and private consultations that I have held, I have gained deeper insights into both the questions and the answers, the analysis and the wisdom behind the issues reflected in these pages. I am inspired by the impressive Jewish value system and its practical guidance, and I yearn to bring these teachings to ever larger numbers.

The book offered here is intended more as a narrative analysis than an expository inquiry. Hence I have omitted this time the footnotes at page-bottom or at chapter-end, while ensuring that many of the quoted sources are identified in the presentation itself. This helps me make the point that no halakhic decisions should be based solely on what is said here. Primary-text sources and rabbinic authorities

3

known to the reader should first be consulted. The reader can also contact me directly by e-mail for additional source citations, literary or otherwise.

I am grateful to members of my family for their warm support and confidence-building. My dear wife Aviva, who set new standards in gracious helpfulness, was joined in this support by our gifted children Rabbi Daniel Zvi and Leah Feldman, Rabbi Jonathan J. and Rachel Feldman, and Rebecca Nechama Feldman. I am likewise grateful to my late brother, Los Angeles Attorney Eliot Bernard (Berel) Feldman, for his consistent encouragement. His lamented passing took place during the final stages of this writing, but his illness had been alleviated, as illness can be, by the pleasure of contemplating the book's potential. I herewith formally dedicate the completed work to his memory.

I thank these and others in the family near and far — including those across the ocean, Mrs. Miriam Cohen in London and Rabbi Meyer and Goldie Fendel in Jerusalem, and closer by, Trude Feldman in Washington — as well as many unnamed teachers, colleagues, and friends, for their edifying words and deeds over the years. They thus share with me in this humble service to God and Torah.

In the practical sphere, I am thankful, too, to the Memorial Foundation for Jewish Culture, for assistance in bringing this to press; to Gil Student and Yashar Books, the excellent instrument of its publication; and to the participants in and supporters of our Jewish Institute of Bioethics, notably Warren and Esther Feldman, Anne Gerad, Kurt Heilbronner, Drs. Benjamin and Miriam Landau, Abe and Sheila Schlussel, and Isaac and Frances Suder. The Institute is always active in disseminating the information, ideals, and value-perspectives set forth in the volume at hand.

Rabbi David M. Feldman

CHAPTER ONE

LIFE IS SACRED

The title of this book sprang forth from a discussion I had been having in a radio interview. The subject was Jewish medical ethics, and, after exploring many of its issues, the interviewer was now ready to conclude the dialogue. He said, "Oh I see what you're saying. You're saying, 'Where there's life, there's hope.'" "No, no," I protested. "I'm not saying anything as unoriginal as that. I'm saying 'Where there's life, there's life. It's precious in and of itself.'" Life is not only precious because there's hope that the disease is curable. Regardless of apparent medical "futility," life is precious because every moment of life has infinite value and intrinsic sanctity, even with no outlook for later, and even in diminished quality.

Such an attitude is profoundly different from one which measures life in terms of its promise or its relative quality, certainly from measuring it in terms of its level of productivity. It's an attitude based on religious principles, but supported strongly by purely secular ones. Life is a gift, as irreplaceable as it is singular and unique. Just as we cannot deprive another human of his or her inalienable life, neither can we do the same to our own life. We cannot surrender it, abuse it, or curtail it. To so regard life as sacred and precious is our best protection against allowing deterioration of the spirit, and

9

our best antidote to the callousness of those who hold life cheap and expendable.

An important motif in the chapters of this book militates against the notion, for instance, that becoming a burden to others must be avoided. The sanctity and inalienability of life also mean that we need not apologize for being alive, that we need not see our own continued existence as a burden to family, to society, to caretakers. Even if we haven't "paid our dues" by caring for others we have not forfeited the right to be a burden. Our own right to life is intrinsic to our humanness, is non-negotiable, and needs no further justification.

Some of the theology and the halakhic directives embodying this view are set forth in the following pages. The presentation here highlights the mechanism of a majestic and pervasive teaching, that of *pikkuach nefesh*. According to this principle, virtually all other *mitzvot* and prohibitions of the Torah are to be set aside if, by doing so, a person can be saved from a threat to life or health. This is an eloquent, and underappreciated, doctrine of the preciousness of life embedded in Jewish law and practice.

"The greatest *mitzvah* is the saving of life," declared R. Shimon ben Tzadok. He lived in fifteenth-century Spain, but he was making explicit what was implicit in the legal rulings of the rabbis in all the centuries and places before and after him. The attitude expressed itself consistently in the prescriptive and descriptive assessments of the Torah's mandate. The attitude elicited disdain—the anti-Semitic philosopher Schopenhauer was said to have based his hatred of the Jews on their indomitable pro-life outlook. And it inspired confidence—in Jewish physicians that they would struggle mightily to heal. R. David Bleich relays a conversation he had with the late R. Yosef Henkin, when the latter had become blind and frail, life having clearly become a burden to him. "How far is one obligated to go in order to prolong life?" the younger rabbi asked him in the form of a halakhic query. Without the slightest hesitation, he answered, "So long as it is possible for a Jew to live, he ought to want to live."

I hesitate to make mention here of the boast of some sponsors of suicide bombing for political reasons, namely that "we love death and you [Israel and the West] love life, so we will vanquish you." The boast is uttered by fringe extremists and is surely not representative, even if it does give us pause. Phrases such as "culture of life" vs. "culture of death" have been seen in many a context in recent days. Most ominous is a phrase like "life unworthy of life," cited by Dr. Paul McHugh of Johns Hopkins University, as the title of a book coming from Germany in 1920. Dr. McHugh laments the culture of death in that awful title and the horrendous public proportions it reached, but his concern is for now— that something like it might weaken the otherwise high resolve of medical caretakers to save life for its own sake.

If saying "where there's life there's hope" sounds "unoriginal," that does not at all detract from its essential truth. More to the point, where there's hope there's life. We ought not to shorten life because we see no hope, and the presence of hope actually adds life. It enhances life when it doesn't lengthen it, by sparing us the depression of forlornness, and it lengthens it medically by the same means. Even when hope ultimately disappoints, it has nurtured and elevated our lives for the duration. Often enough, hope does more: It advances therapeutic progress by its benign effect. This fact, too, is reflected in the details of the halakhic and philosophic motifs of the presentation herein. The power and potential of the *pikkuach nefesh* provisions come from both the affirmation of life and the exaltation of hope.

Hope's healing power in situations of ordinary stress, and in those of medical crisis, has been effectively set forth in recent books. *The Power of Hope* by Rabbi Maurice Lamm calls hope "the essential ingredient in life and love" and demonstrates its positive and beneficent effect. Dr. Jerome Groopman, in *The Anatomy of Hope*, celebrates the role of hope at life's critical junctures. The book keeps clear of fostering false hope, but encourages realistic hope that carries us through to the good outcome.

That life itself has infinite value is true in the technical legal sense, as we hear in the text of the *Minchat Chinnukh*, the commentary to a fundamental exposition of biblical precepts. That source declares: "Even if the Prophet Elijah himself were to tell us that a given individual has only a few minutes to live, the Torah does not differentiate between one who kills a child who otherwise might live for many years, and one who kills a 100-year-old person with only a limited life expectancy. Even if the victim were about to die anyway, the act is the same one of homicide because life has been destroyed, if only by a second."

The thesis of this book is the positive side of that coin, that life itself has infinite value, unrelated to any consideration of circumstances or of outcome. This theological affirmation is expressed in the legal provisions of Jewish law and practice, in a manner both impressive and unequivocal. Its message is that life is a precious gift even without hope for future relief or future survival, and that the presence of hope is a healing companion.

I am proud of the salutation *"l'chayyim,"* expressing the Jewish affirmation of life and inspiration to live, and confidently urge it on those who must make difficult decisions. Some thinkers disdain the approach, at least in its extremes, as mere "vitalism," a kind of mindless respect for any human life, even of little or no quality. The point of *"l'chayyim"* is a more profound sanctification of life. It issues from an abhorrence of causing a death, or of callous cheapening of life's value and, before that, it issues from awesome reverence for the image of God within us. It issues from a loyalty to faith in the transcendence of life over all that life presents, good and bad.

We are bidden *"uvacharta ba-chayyim,* you shall choose life." Our basic supplication at High Holy Day time is *"zokhreinu l'chayyim,* remember us unto life," a prayer which we direct to the Author of life, Who is "*chafetz ba-chayyim*," the God Who endorses life, in spite of enormous challenges to the very idea. And if one is tempted to claim that these sentiments refer on some level to eternal life, to life in the next world, it is good to consider the standard expression of gratitude for life here and now and all by itself. Our inspiring culture of life thanks God "*she-hecheyanu v'kiyy'manu v'higgiyanu la-z'man ha-zeh*, Who hast kept us in life, sustained us, and brought us to this time." That's enough to ask for.

Where there's life there's hope, and where there's hope there's life, and where there's nothing but life there's life, which is everything.

CHAPTER TWO

SAVING LIFE AND HEALTH

W hat this chapter title addresses is the basic *mitzvah* of rescuing someone in apparent danger. The biblical text (Leviticus 19:16) "Do not stand (idly) by the blood of your neighbor" is applied as follows by the Talmud (*Sanhedrin* 73a): Do not stand and watch with indifference when your fellowman is in mortal danger through drowning, or attacked by wild animals, or by marauders, without hastening to attempt his rescue. The Talmud here, however, also exempts one from doing so if his or her own life would be endangered by the attempt. But there is another *mitzvah* that is less obvious and also less threatening, and a much clearer illustration of the distinctive ethic of Jewish law and practice.

The keystone principle that translates Judaism's reverence for life into action is called *pikkuach nefesh*, the saving of life and health. Literally, the words happen to mean "removal of a life [from harm's way]." The slightly unusual phrasing ties the principle to its signal example in the Talmud (*Yoma* 81a), which speaks of removal of a victim from the debris of a collapsed building on the Sabbath. We are told to "set aside" the Sabbath and strive to extricate the victim, to determine if he or she is still alive (the criteria here give us the indicia of death; see Chapter Seven) and to revive the victim. The principle is now established that steps must be taken to forestall a perceived threat to one's life or health, even when other issues might seem to take precedence, and even when the saving is only for *chayyei sha'ah*, for momentary life. It is not a voluntary or permissive act, but an imperative—a *mitzvah* in the sense of an obligation—that takes first place in the hierarchy of values to be acted upon, setting aside any restrictions or duties of the moment.

The principle is announced boldly in the Talmud's formulation: *"ein l'kha davar ha-omed bif'nei pikkuach nefesh,* nothing should stand in the way of saving a life" (*Yoma* 82a). Three areas of exception will be listed below, but for all other ritual matters of the Sabbath, Yom Kippur, the dietary laws, and more, the principle stands firm.

On what did the Rabbis of the Talmud base this emphatic and unanimous teaching? Some sample prooftexts:

"How do we know that removal of a threat to life sets aside the Sabbath?" the Talmud asks (*Yoma* 85b). 1) Rabbi Simon ben Menassia answers: "We are told: 'You shall keep the Sabbath, for it is holy unto you' (Exodus 31:13). That means, 'unto you' is the Sabbath given over, but you are not given over to the Sabbath." 2) Rabbi Nathan: "We are told: 'The people of Israel shall keep the Sabbath, to observe the Sabbath throughout their generations' (Exodus 31:16). That means, [if necessary] violate one Sabbath in order to [stay alive] and observe many Sabbaths [thereafter]." 3) Rabbi Judah in the name of Rabbi Samuel: "We are told: 'Keep My commandments and ordinances, which if a man do them he will live by them' (Leviticus 18:5). That means, live by them and not die because of them."

There is much to say, historically and legally, about each of these exegetical teachings. The first one figures in a New Testament narrative, where Mark (2:27) quotes Jesus as defending his acts of public healing on the Sabbath. For this, he cites the rabbinic teaching, "The Sabbath is given to man, not man to the Sabbath." And, centuries earlier, the Maccabbees demonstrated, in their war against the Greek Syrians, that keeping the Sabbath should not render them indefensible in the face of enemy attack

The second exegetical point has implications for basic orientation to life. Are we otherworldly or thisworldly? Is the focus of religious efforts this world or the next? In an otherworldly orientation, it would not matter much if one were to die in observing the Sabbath. His reward would be condign in the next world. But in the thisworldly attitude of the Talmudic passage, the goal is to preserve life, to remain alive here on earth for the allotted time, to "stick around" so as to "keep many Sabbaths."

The third derivation gives us the principle and, at the same time, the exceptions thereto. "[Do] not die because of them"—except, that is, in the case of one of the three cardinal sins. Rather die, rather undergo martyrdom, than transgress the sin of murder, of idolatry, or of adultery-incest. For all other coerced violations of the Torah, sins of commission or of omission, *"ya'avor v'al yehareg,* let one transgress rather than be killed." But not for these three. If one is asked to murder (the innocent, as opposed to killing, in self-defense, the no-longer innocent attacker), then *yehareg v'al ya'avor,* let him be killed rather than transgress the overriding commandment "Thou shalt not murder." Or, if one is asked to bow publicly to idols, as were Hannah and her seven sons in the days of the Maccabbees, then one must accept martyrdom, as they did. Lastly, the sin of gross sexual immorality is serious enough to require martyrdom instead.

Barring these three, when observance of say, the Sabbath or Yom Kippur or any ritual or other commandment (see on), entails a threat to one's life or health, then such a threat "sets aside the entire Torah." And if these three seem too many or too harsh, the Talmud records the rule as a delimitation, not a recommendation. Evidently, people were ready to martyr themselves for lesser challenges; so, during the Hadrianic persecutions, the Rabbis, in a synod "in the upper chambers of the house of Nitza in Lydda" (*Sanhedrin* 74a), solemnly ruled that only in these three situations may such extreme steps be taken.

The principle of physical safety emerges uncontested in an entirely different context, one where the relationship between spiritual and physical wellbeing is defined. This is reflected in the legal precept enunciated elsewhere in the Talmud (*Chullin* 9a): "*Chamira sakkanta me'issura*," meaning "That which is [physically/medically] dangerous is more to be avoided than the [ritually] forbidden." The matter of infant circumcision also illustrates the principle: the Torah ordains that the *b'rit* take place on "the eighth day," meaning with no postponement, even if the eighth day falls on the Sabbath or Yom Kippur. Only health considerations, such as symptoms of jaundice, allow and require postponement—on the judgment of the mohel, whose opinion will be even more cautious than that of the medical staff.

Though comparisons are invidious, and competitiveness is unworthy, the boldness of the general principle can best be seen by a look, for example, at teachings of Jehovah's Witnesses. That religious group shares the Hebrew Bible, the so-called Old Testament, as a textual source of many of its practices, notably Leviticus 7:26 "Do not eat the blood." The rabbinic tradition specifies that "eating" refers only to the usual manner of doing so,

not, say, through intravenous infusion. The latter is assumed to be permitted, the former forbidden. But the
doctrine of *pikkuach nefesh* teaches that even eating blood
in the normal manner would be permissible to save a
human life. For less than life-saving reasons, we must
take pains to remove every bit of forbidden blood, a pre-
requisite in the preparation of kosher food. But the power
of *pikkuach nefesh* makes clear that saving life overrides
even this serious prohibition. For devotees of the Witnesses, martyrdom must be chosen rather than ingestion
of blood in any manner, or for any reason.

The basic doctrine has its classic illustration in the
paradigmatic example of the Yom Kippur Fast. As opposed to other fast days on the Jewish calendar which are
rabbinically ordained—such as Tishah B'Av, commemo-
rating the destruction of the Temple in Jerusalem in 586
BCE and in 70 CE, and other such fasts—Yom Kippur is
biblical, and the fast is fundamental to its observance. Yet,
in keeping with all the above, any threat to a person's
health occasioned by fasting means that it becomes one's
mitzvah to break the fast and eat rather than to abstain.
The *mitzvah* of sustaining health overrides that of the fast,
and one must take adequate nutriment. Of course, one is
not to feast, only to take what is minimally necessary to
stay in health.* The regimen has been interpreted to
mean, as well, that if medications are necessary, but require accompanying liquid to help them function, then

---

* R. Chayyim Brisker famously ruled otherwise, that staying too
close to the minimum may be countertherapeutic. He defended this
ruling by explaining "I am not being lenient with regard to the restrictions of Yom Kippur. I am being strict with regard to the requirements of *pikkuach nefesh!*"

the liquid is also mandated. If chemotherapy must continue uninterrupted, and if food is required so that it help rather than harm, then food must accompany the treatment.

What about the malingerer or the hypochondriac, who only thinks he needs to eat? No such thing. In the Talmud's further discussion of the teaching, the patient is supreme, the doctor second in line. "One who feels ill on Yom Kippur is given to eat on the advice of the physician" (*Yoma* 83a) is the rule. What if the physician deems him ill but the patient feels himself strong enough to fast? We follow the physician, we cause him to eat, because this is risky or foolish piety. What if, on the other hand, the physician declares him well enough to fast, but the patient doesn't think so? Then we listen to the patient rather than to the doctor—for, as implied in the Scriptural verse, "The heart knoweth its own bitterness" (Proverbs 14:10). The subjective component is real. Perceived danger is also danger in this context.

Which leads us to broaden further an already wide principle. Instead of saying "A threat to life sets aside the entire Torah," we need to re-state that as "A possible threat to life sets aside the entire Torah," or, as the Talmud indeed puts it, *safek pikkuach nefesh docheh kol ha-Torah*. After all, none of us is equipped to be an instant diagnostician, nor can the seriousness of any threat be immediately verified. Obviously, then, we must avert the threat before it becomes real. In the classic example, if a pregnant woman experiences labor pains in the synagogue on the Sabbath or Yom Kippur, she must be transported hurriedly to the hospital. If she then finds the labor pains were false labor pains, then—better safe than sorry.

To carry the matter further, we are taught not only not to wait for certainty, but not to wait at all. "The diligent one [*ha-zariz*]," says the Talmud, that is, the one who is quick and unhesitant in bringing relief for a threat, "is praiseworthy," because he or she may have saved a life. Moreover, other considerations should be ignored so that they not cause one to hesitate. For example, there are certain deeds forbidden to a Jew on the Sabbath, but not of course to a non-Jew, and so one might have thought to wait for the helpful non-Jew to perform them. Ordinarily so, but not here. Rushing someone to a hospital or to a place of relief should not await the help of non-Jews in order to avoid Sabbath violations—this can cause delay. Even if it does not cause delay, onlookers may wrongly conclude that the Torah does not command the Sabbath to be set aside forthwith for life-saving work.

Nor should we leave the rescue to under-age children who would not technically be bound by the Sabbath restrictions. In the Talmud's continuing words: "This (rescue work) should be done only by *gedolei Yisrael*," which is understood by some as "adult Jews," but which Maimonides translates literally as "the great ones of Israel," meaning even the more learned and respected, the better to make the point. Hence, the *Hatzalah* agencies, the Orthodox volunteer ambulance groups, make sure that a recognizably observant (even bearded) Jewish emergency worker accompanies the patient to the hospital. This again is to demonstrate that life-saving efforts are not a grudging concession of the law or an attempt to work around it, but an affirmative commandment.

The Talmud quoted so often here is the *Bavli*, the Babylonian recension of rabbinic discussion over the centuries, as opposed to the *Yerushalmi*, the Palestinian record of parallel discussions in the Land of Israel. The latter came to its close earlier than the former; the former is the more extensive and authoritative. The version of the *Yerushalmi* in its treatment of this matter deserves to be cited. After insisting on diligence and speed in setting the rescue in motion, and holding the hesitant guilty of possible bloodshed, the *Yerushalmi* goes on to assign blame for any delay to the very *rabbi* who is consulted—the one who could have prevented delay if he would have taught the people clearly in advance that it's wrong to hesitate!

But hesitate we will, and hence the active example of the rabbi is important. A page from modern Hebrew literature makes vivid a recent historical demonstration of this principle of *pikkuach nefesh* and the role of the rabbi in bringing it about. Y. L. Peretz, a novelist of a half-century ago, tells the story of how the illustrious Rabbi Israel Salanter acted publicly and dramatically in a situation of crisis in the nineteenth century. Alluding to the Talmud's discussion of the rule in the Mishnah for Grace After Meals for *sh'loshah she-ach'lu*, or three who ate together, Peretz takes the title of that Talmudic chapter "Three Who Ate" and makes it the title of his story as well. He relates the circumstances of the spread of cholera at that time and place. It's Yom Kippur and the beloved Rabbi Salanter has told his congregation that they must break their fast in order to maintain resistance to the plague. They hesitate; perhaps the plague will pass them by, perhaps they will be strong enough to resist it even while fasting. The rabbi saw no alternative. He went and brought and gave food—to the cantor, the sexton, and himself. These were "three who ate"—demonstratively—in order to teach by their unequivocal action what religious law demanded for that moment.

This is matched by a surreal story, one that elaborates poignantly on the idea that taking life-saving steps is not an evasion but a fulfillment of commandment: Eating bread on Passover is another fundamental prohibition in Judaism. Only unleavened bread, *matzah*, may be eaten, and at the Seder night the obligatory consumption thereof is preceded by the blessing uttered before performing such a ritual act—"Blessed art Thou, Lord our God, Sovereign of the Universe, who hast sanctified us by Thy commandments, and commanded us concerning the eating of *matzah*." Among the stories of religious faith and heroism emerging from the awful Holocaust days is a particular incident told of Jewish death-camp inmates. These hapless individuals, upon finding and taking up a discarded morsel of bread on Passover that might keep them alive another day, summoned the strength to recite first "…hast sanctified us by Thy commandments and commanded us concerning preservation of life and health."

The remarkable principle gets better. Not only are we to stand clear of a threat to life and health, and not only of a possible threat, but also—of a psychological threat. This dimension of the principle has its central example in the Mishnah itself, where the subject is childbirth on the Sabbath (*Shabbat* 128b). The woman in labor asks the doctor to kindle additional light so that he can better minister to her. But the doctor responds: There is sufficient light; I can see fine. She insists on more light. The ruling is given that the doctor must kindle more light for her sake, "to set her mind at ease." To appreciate the ruling's significance, we must remember that this was established in pre-electricity days, when light meant actual fire. Kindling fire on the Sabbath is a serious Biblical violation, as possibly opposed to the derivative extension thereof, namely closing an electric circuit. But "to set her mind at ease," so that childbirth proceed safely, we must certainly activate our exalted principle by overriding a prohibition clearly on the Biblical level.

To remove any doubt about the psychological dimension—and to carry forward its then-novel insights for the mind-body connection—the Talmud makes it explicit in another passage (*Yoma* 82). *Teruf da'at*, a threat to mental equilibrium, is to be treated like *pikkuach nefesh*, a threat to one's physical life. The authoritative Nachmanides (Ramban, the rabbi-physician of a half-century later than his colleague Maimonides, Rambam) spells out what this means in his medical-halakhic work, *Torat haAdam*: Just as measures in violation of ritual law may be taken for physical threats, so may they be taken for mental ones. A piquant example comes from a late seventeenth-century respondent: A certain nonkosher soup was reputed to have therapeutic properties; one person insisted he would go out of his mind unless he had some. R. Israel Meir Mizrachi, noting that serious danger to mental health is tantamount to a risk to one's physical wellbeing, issued a permissive ruling where that was indeed the case, to allow the forbidden soup to save sanity! Mental health is important to the *pikkuach nefesh* of self-protection; hence when a genuine threat to sanity presented itself, some would permit what would maintain it, as a safeguard against self-destructive action. Some would allow concessions to protect sanity for its own sake.

This approach was, in fact, also taken in the case of more common, or more serious, needs—such as abortion. In 1913, R. Mordecai Winkler was asked if abortion could be permitted to a woman whose mental health was threatened by her ongoing pregnancy. Among other arguments in response, he wrote:

"Mental-health risk has been definitely equated to physical-health risk (in Jewish law). This woman, who is in danger of losing her mental health if the pregnancy continues, would accordingly qualify." Now generally, the warrant for abortion is predicated on the welfare of the mother and not the condition of the fetus. There is no permission to abort because of fear that the fetus may be defective; for in that case the consensus of rabbinic opinion is that one cannot know "the secrets of God," or what would eventuate with the child. But where there is danger in the here and now to the mother, she, being an actual rather than a potential person, deserves all the consideration to prevent an untoward outcome, whether physical or mental.

The case of a Tay-Sachs conception might seem different, since the pregnancy will do her no physical or mental harm. But the prospect of giving birth to a child doomed to die in infancy gives her extreme mental anguish. Accordingly, some rabbinic authorities do say no to an abortion for Tay-Sachs, because that's a fetal consideration, not a maternal one. Others say, the fact of her mental anguish transforms the case from a fetal to a maternal matter, and abortion should be permitted—here and in other cases where mental anguish is a real factor. And it is important to note here what will be said in the later chapter on the subject of abortion: In the case of genuine physical hazard, the woman has no "choice" of abortion or not. The principle of *pikkuach nefesh* mandates that she terminate the pregnancy, "because her life comes first."

Contraception, too, can be brought forth as an example, though that does take us back for a moment to physical rather than psychological considerations. There is extensive discussion in the Talmud of both methods of and reasons for contraception. But the *locus classicus* of the various legal opinions on the matter (*Yevamot* 12b) actually centers on whether women who may need protection are ever permitted to do without it. If pregnancy is contraindicated, and the contraceptive methods available seem onanistic and unacceptable, you might conclude that therefore sexual abstinence in marriage is the recommended alternative. The discussion yields a different conclusion: Abstinence is wrong, but the woman's physical wellbeing must be safeguarded. We solve the dilemma by overcoming as best we can the objections to contraception or contraceptive means, and affirming the primacy of marital relations alongside the protection of her health.

One could go further and point out that standard pregnancy itself brings the woman to a state of risk. It admittedly does, but the risk has been called "normative" and obviously worth taking. This can explain a curious fact in the understanding of the first commandment of the Torah, namely *"p'ru ur'vu*, be fruitful and multiply." The curious fact is that the Mishnah and Talmud see this *mitzvah* as applying to the man and not the woman. Not the woman? How can the man perform the *mitzvah* without her? The answer is that his is the *mitzvah* in the sense of obligation, hers in the sense of privilege. The best explanation of this anomaly comes from R. Meir Simcha Ha-Kohen of Dvinsk, of the early twentieth century, in his Bible commentary (to Gen. 1:28) called *Meshekh Chokhmah*. He cites the verse chanted by the congregation when the Torah Scroll is brought out for public reading, namely "Its ways are ways of pleasantness and all its paths are peace" (Proverbs 3:17). Since the Torah's ways are pleasant and not cruel, how could the Torah command a woman to enter pregnancy, thus inviting a state of possible risk and likely pain in childbirth, not to mention discomfort and morning sickness? The command therefore devolves upon the man—for whom the procreative act bears no risk or pain—impelling him to use sexuality responsibly. It allows the woman the privilege of expressing her maternal instinct and choosing to accept the risk and pain.

Threat to life, possible threat to life, threat to mental wellbeing as well as physical—a powerful and noble principle, but we may broaden the principle still further. This would embrace the caretakers and emphasize their obligation, as well, to set aside the Torah and do what is helpful to the person threatened, whether this help is physical or psychological. Hence, regarding the woman in the above case who feels labor pains at the height of Yom Kippur services in the Synagogue and must be rushed to the hospital without delay, her husband, too, must violate the restrictions of the day and accompany her in the ambulance to the hospital. Why is he permitted and encouraged to do so? Though he may have not a modicum of midwifery skill, he "holds her hand"—that is, he offers a husband's reassurance and moral support, psychological elements that contribute greatly to the medical effort. In his absence from the scene, this would apply to other bystanders, or even a patient's advocate, whose support can be significant.

CHAPTER THREE

MORE ON
PIKKUACH NEFESH

There is much more to be said in illustration of this important principle and its application.

Picture the doctor himself comfortably ensconced with his family around the Sabbath table, when he is summoned to the bedside of a patient far away. Must he leave his home in say, New Jersey, and travel to Manhattan in response to the call, all this in obedience to the imperative of *pikkuach nefesh* for a faraway patient in emergent need? He could correctly demur by reminding the patient that Manhattan is not without its many doctors, and there should be no need for him to break many rules of the Sabbath just to please the caller. But our noble rule says otherwise. If this doctor and that patient have a bond of trust, then it's this doctor who has the best chance of therapeutic success, and the Sabbath must be set aside to bring the two together. And it's not the doctor's greater professional expertise that promises the success, but the psychological factor of the bond of trust and confidence between them.

Now the harder question: May the doctor return to his home after treating the patient, the emergency now having passed? Or does he have to remain in Manhattan until the Sabbath is over? It may not be just "the Sabbath," but it could be a two-day religious festival, or two days attached to a Sabbath for a three-day non-traveling chunk of time. Does he have to remain one, two or three days away from his family and his life and be anchored "in exile" for all that time? The answer is no. He may return home after his ministrations are finished, though the Sabbath, or more, is still with us. But why? The crisis is finished, so what permits him to violate the Sabbath now?

The answer is admittedly psychological. He may return on the Sabbath and Yom Tov, so that he should not hesitate to make the trip the next time he is called. He must not be tempted to hide behind rationalizations—for example, that he is not *really* needed. R. Mosheh Feinstein (*Iggerot Mosheh, Orach Chayyim* 4:80) compares the fear of rationalization in this context with that in other Talmudic provisions, and sees it as causing the doctor wrongly to hesitate. To forestall the hesitation, he broadly permitted the return the same day, while R. Shlomoh Zalman Auerbach (*Minchat Shlomoh* 1:8) limited the extent of the permissible to non-biblical prohibitions where possible. According to both authorities, clearly *pikkuach nefesh* goes further in this example of the doctor's return on Shabbat—it allows violations now that would prevent subconscious rationalizing, and harmful hesitation, next time.

We must be careful not to extrapolate from this ruling a license for other future-oriented activity. True, we may, for example, violate the Sabbath by cooking what's needed for a seriously ill person. But the parameters of *pikkuach nefesh* specifically

exclude doing so on the Sabbath for what the patient may not need until the next day. Even with
regard to immediate need, the *halakhah* provides for
varying categories of "dangerously ill," "not-
dangerously ill," and "bearably ill," prescribing
what may or may not be done in each of these
cases. And, after preparing ourselves not to hesitate, we must still distinguish between levels of
likelihood. For the relevant paradigm in this category we go far afield, to a Mishnaic teaching with
regard to the Silent Prayer. In prescribing proper
demeanor for the recitation of this central prayer,
the Talmud (*Berakhot* 33a) allows one to break his
worshipful posture and interrupt his praying only
to ward off an approaching scorpion—but not a
snake! The snake, commentaries explain, is more
dangerous only if it bites, but it may not bite;
while the scorpion more likely will. The nineteenth-century authority Rabbi Jacob Ettlinger is
thus led to draw a distinction, in his *Responsa Bin-
yan Tziyyon,* for *pikkuach nefesh* in the face of a present and immediate or likely danger, on the one
hand, and a potential but less likely danger, on the
other.

This, incidentally, takes us in a new direction,
to another important issue. What about avoiding a
threat to the physician from tending a sick patient? The question, and R. Ettlinger's distinction,
were brought into play in connection with the
scourge of AIDS. Since the infection can be con-
tracted by the attending physician, is he or she allowed to forget their own *pikkuach nefesh* in order

to relieve the threat facing the patient? Historically, doctors have been heroic in doing just that,
in putting their lives and wellbeing on the line in
order to relieve the patient's condition. Why, now,
should the threat of AIDS contamination be any
different? In response, it was argued that treating
small pox, for example, brings one into likely but
not necessarily fatal danger, while treating AIDS
would subject one to unlikely but fatal contagion.
It is rendered more unlikely by avoiding any exchange of or exposure to fluids and assuring that
properly sterile safeguards are in place.

There remains still another application of our
principle, an application that is admittedly psychological but nonetheless profound. One's essential will to live can be undermined by the loss
of faith or hope; death can in fact be hastened by
giving up the struggle too soon. This insight is reflected in the Talmudic provision that the *viddui*,
the confession, of a terminally ill person should
not capitulate to hopelessness and assume the
worst. One's confession should not contain words
like, "God, I am about to die. Please forgive my
sins and grant me a share in the World to Come,
etc." To say even that much surrenders the will to
live. What should instead be uttered is something
like, "God, grant me healing. If not, then forgive
my sins, etc." This guidance has bearing on the
question of whether the doctor should be allowed
to reveal to the patient the full seriousness of his
or her condition. The family has its need to know,
but the patient's survival can actually be adversely

affected by the doctor's ready candor or pessimism.

The patient's wellbeing can certainly be affected by starkly yielding to predictions of imminent death. This led to an uncommon discussion between two contemporary rabbinic authorities, in written correspondence between them.* One suggested that the doctor's frankness in leveling with the patient might be a favor, in that it will impel the patient to proceed to his death-bed repentance. Repentance is a *mitzvah* which one might otherwise have omitted by postponement, thinking that there is still time for that. The second rabbi—his name was R. Aaron Zaslansky—referred to the clear statement in his book: Final repentance may indeed be a *mitzvah*, he wrote, but are we not told to "set aside" every *mitzvah* to save even momentary life? This demand of *pikkuach nefesh* says that life should not be defeated even by psychological danger. Set aside the *mitzvah* of confession so that death not be hastened by surrender to harsh and unbending prognoses.

I make bold to claim that our principle of *pikkuach nefesh* has its influence in still another, unexpected area. It can answer the puzzle of Judaism's attitude to capital punishment. The pervasive emphasis in the Torah on the pursuit of justice makes allowance for our natural tendency to bias, and asks that the bias, if there is to be such, be enlisted

---

* A printed copy of this exchange was made available by R. Ya'akov Neuburger.

in favor of the accused. To begin with, the Biblical directives *"v'shaf'tu ha-edah,* the community shall judge..." and *"v'hitzillu ha-edah,* the community shall save [the accused]..." (Numbers 35:24, 25) look descriptive of a routine process. In the Talmud, however, the latter phrase "...and the community shall save..." is understood to be prescriptive—to direct us, when possible, to strive for acquittal when judging. This is the source of the humanitarian idea of being vigorous in defense of the accused.

But there's more. Obviously, the stern judgment, *"mot yamut,* he shall surely die" is found so often in Scripture, making us wonder at the rabbinic approach. We must wonder at the Mishnaic citation of the proud words of R. Tarfon and R. Akiva, that "If we had been members of the Sanhedrin, there would never be an instance of capital execution" on our watch (Talmud, *Makkot* 7a). To which R. Simon ben Gamaliel rejoined: Failure to implement capital punishment when called for would only "increase bloodshed in Israel" because of the lawlessness it would encourage.

In fact, the requirements necessary to secure a penalty of death were made so exacting—two witnesses are needed to testify not only that they saw the accused commit the crime, but also that they gave him formal warning, and more, that he acknowledged the warning and proceeded to defy it—so exacting that it was well-nigh impossible for a capital conviction ever to happen. The result is a radical departure in the Talmud from the Bible's apparently freer attitude to capital punishment. What could justify this departure? On one level, the answer can be the rabbis' awareness that, in the initial instance in Genesis (2:17) of "ye shall surely die," it was addressed to Adam and Eve, threatening them with death if they ate from the forbidden fruit in the Garden of Eden. But when they did transgress, they were not executed, but merely banished from the Garden.

This means, one could say, that the Bible's "bark is worse than its bite," and that such threats are needed as a probable deterrent to crime. When it comes to execution, however, so many extenuating factors need to be considered. The main extenuating factor in the human court is the possibility of error by the human prosecutor. As the Talmud reminds us elsewhere, when the judge makes an error in a monetary judgment, that error can always be rectified when the truth emerges. In a capital case, a life has been taken and the error is irreversible. So the doctrine of *pikkuach nefesh* means that we have a mandate to save life in one more sphere, to save life also against the possibility of human error.

I conclude these two chapters on the doctrine of *pikkuach nefesh* by citing the remarkable statement by Maimonides. It is a conclusion to his summary of this category of suspension of the law, in a truly legal context, but now with a more theological and humane reflection. He writes (*Hilkhot Shabbat* 2:3): We are commanded to set aside the Torah in these instances of threat to life, because

"the Torah's provisions are not acts of vindictiveness (*n'kamah*) against the world, but an instrument of mercy and kindness and wholeness
(peace) for the world."

This is a striking and bold formulation. He explains: The Torah sets forth laws to guide us, but
not to mislead us; hence we are protected by the
verse (Lev. 18:5) that presents the commandments
as given to us "*va-chai bahem*, that one... live by
them," not die because of them. This translates
into the positive imperative of *pikkuach nefesh*,
wherein the Torah becomes a blueprint by which
life may be enhanced and not stunted.

The presence of the word *olam* ("the world")
twice in the statement by Maimonides suggests a
kind of universalism, that although the ritual prohibitions of the Sabbath devolve primarily on the
Jewish people, the *mitzvah* to set them aside and
save life—though this is inferred not by Maimonides but by a consensus of subsequent authorities—extends as well to rescuing non-Jews in life-
threatening situations, particularly given today's
expectations of universal medical treatment. The
oft-quoted maxim that "he who saves a single life
saves a whole world" (*Sanhedrin* 37a, the text as in
most manuscripts) is wondrous in its teaching that
when an individual loses his life he or she loses
the ability to perceive or interact with the whole
world. Its context is the uplifting passage in the
Talmud that reflects on why man was created as
an individual (Adam), rather than in groups or
races. In order, explains the Talmud, that no one

claim superiority over others by virtue of descent from a supposedly superior group. Considering the significance of each individual, then, "whoever destroys a single life destroys a whole world, and whoever saves a single life saves a whole world."

Postcript: In the Spring 1994 issue of *The Pharos*, a medical journal, Dr. Michael Farbowitz has an article entitled "The Responsibility of the Jewish Physician in Jewish Law." He addresses the problem of desecration of the Sabbath by a Jewish physician in order to save the health or life of a non-Jewish patient, to whom the Sabbath has no meaning (remembering "Violate for him this Sabbath so that he may live to keep many Sabbaths"). Why should this be permitted? In answer, he says it had been assumed that the Jewish physician should do so, for at least social or political reasons (*"mi-shum eivah"*), but the author tells us that "the Rav," R. Joseph B. Soloveitchik, responded otherwise to this question by R. Shlomo Riskin, as the latter testified in a public lecture in 1990. The Rav reminded us that having been created in the image of God is a basic reason for our affirmation of life. And since gentiles are equally created in the image of God, said the Rav, this is proper and sufficient reason to suspend our Sabbath to save the gentile's life or health.

CHAPTER FOUR

NATALISM AND REPRODUCTIVE TECHNOLOGY

"Pronatalist" is a contemporary word, but it describes well the classic Jewish tradition on childbirth. Procreation is counted as a positive *mitzvah*, given pride of place at the top of rabbinic lists of biblical commandments. *P'ru ur'vu* ("be fruitful and multiply") in the first chapter of Genesis is taken as a blessing to other creatures, whereas to humans it is a command to reproduce. The commentaries explain this difference on its own terms, and as negating anti-procreative or celibate views in other cultures. More than the blessing, the command is needed because man, created in the image of God, might seek to devote himself entirely to the spiritual and intellectual, and neglect the material and physical. Alternatively, since only man is aware of the consequences of his sexual activity, he might seek to avoid the attendant responsibilities of childbirth while indulging his sexual drive. Yet another rabbinic comment observes that throughout Genesis 1, the statement "The Lord saw that it was good" is repeated for each element of creation. With man, the Lord said more, "It is not good that man should be alone." Only that which can endure is good; if man does not procreate he will not endure.

Nor will God Himself endure without us to acknowledge Him: "He who does not engage in procreation diminishes the Divine image," the Talmud declares. Hence, the verse "for in the image of God has He created man" (Gen. 9:6) is immediately followed by a second "be fruitful and multiply." More, a later verse (17:7) introduces the Lord Who will be "thy God and [that] of thy descendants after thee." But "if there are no 'descendants after thee,'" demands the Talmud, "upon whom will the Divine Presence rest? Upon sticks and stones?" Without human descendants, there is no one to worship God. Without the physical body there is no soul.

In spelling out the details of this commandment, the rabbis set forth the *halakhah* of birth control by requiring that a couple at least replace itself, that is, give birth to at least a son and a daughter. Having either several sons or several daughters does not yet fulfill the commandment. But, "grandchildren are like children," so parents with children of one gender can be comforted that they have a second chance with the grandchildren. And since two children is the minimum, remaining with that number, according to Tosafot (*Bava Batra* 60b), could lead to national extinction. Infant mortality, or uncertainty if the offspring themselves will be viable persons or parents, requires that more than the minimum be sired.

Adding to the biblically ordained minimum, therefore, is the rabbinic dimension of the *mitzvah*, which was called, in brief, *lashevet* or *la-erev*. The first comes from the verse in Isaiah 45:18: "Not for void did He create the world, but for habitation

[*lashevet*] did He form it." The second is from Ec-
clesiastes 11:6: "In the morning sow thy seed, and
in the evening [*la-erev*] do not withhold thy hand
[from continuing to sow], for you know not which
will succeed, this or that, or whether they shall
both alike be good." This construction is now part
of the *mitzvah*. Conceptually as well as legally, the
Jewish pro-natalist stance perceives barreness or
infertility as a condition actively to be remedied,
no less than other kinds of illness or pathology.

Another technical requirement of Jewish law
places the responsibility for procreation on the
man rather than on the woman, though of course
it takes both to fulfill the *mitzvah*. This curious law
may have its basis in the theoretical permissibility
of polygamy, or polygyny as opposed to polyan-
dry, whereby a man could marry more than one
wife. This "double standard" would at least make
known both the paternity and maternity of the
children, which the alternatives would not, while
monogamy was seen to be more ethical as well as
more practical. But in marriage of any kind, the
sex-role difference is associated with the latter
part of "Be fruitful and multiply, fill the earth and
conquer it"—that is, he, being the more aggressive
of the two, must worry about procreation,
whereas she, the more passive and coy, should not
have to "go seeking in the marketplace." These
anthropological reasons are improved upon by the
suggestion of a recent rabbinic scholar and Bible
commentator, R. Meir Simchah of Dvinsk (d.
1927), whom we quoted above in Chapter 2. He

writes: Both the pain and the risk of childbearing are borne by the woman, not the man. Since the Torah is not only fair but "its ways are ways of pleasantness and all its paths are peace" (Prov. 3:17), the Torah could not in fairness command a woman to undergo pain and risk; this must be her own choice. For the man, however, exposed to neither pain nor risk, there is the command and the responsibility to fulfill the command.

It goes without saying that attitudes to procreation were not shaped or nurtured through law alone. Abraham protests to God (Gen. 15:2): "What canst Thou give me, seeing that I go childless?" The anguish of the barren woman is a recurrent theme in the Bible and beyond. The most cherished blessing, on the other hand, is fecundity, which is exemplified idyllically in the Psalmist's (Ps. 128) image of one whose "wife is a fruitful vine" and whose "children are as olive plants around the table" and whose ultimate satisfaction is the sight of "children [born] to thy children." The natural desire to overcome barrenness is assumed. Historical circumstances of frequent massacres and forced conversions, with their resulting decimation of Jewish communities, served to elicit compensatory tendencies and to strengthen the procreative impulse. The spoken or unspoken sentiment is to make up for the physical losses of the European Holocaust and the spiritual losses of assimilation. This plays a part in attitudes to abortion as well.

The people's will to replenish its depleted ranks gave added dimension to the instinctive yearning for offspring. Leaders of today are, in fact, urging Jewish families to add a *"mitzvah child"* to the numbers otherwise intended. The attitude contrasts with other reactions to reality; it contrasts, for example, with the anti-procreational stand, born of despair, taken by the first-century Gnostics, the fifth-century Manichees, or the twelfth-century Cathars, who taught and lived by the teaching that procreation is to be avoided in an evil world. On the other hand, avoiding procreation for the benefit of the world is a contemporary issue, acknowledged by the Jewish community as an ethical concern in regard to available resources. The earth's ecology and the effect on human wellbeing of the depletion of finite resources are a Jewish concern as well. Except that, constituting less than one percent of the world's population, the Jewish people could double its present numbers without affecting the world's problems of space and resources, and without undermining the claimed objectives of "zero population growth." Replacing our losses does not upset the numerical balance; it merely keeps us alive. Other minorities should similarly be allowed to maintain their numbers. Our aspirations, as reflected in the daily Prayer Book, are not that we outnumber or overtake the world, but only that "the remnant of the People of Israel be preserved."

In the face of a precarious future—to return to internal history—procreation is essentially an act of faith. Adverse economic or political realities were defied by maternal and religious imperatives. But medical considerations can constitute a risk we are forbidden to take. Here the imperious but exalted principle of *pikkuach nefesh* orders the woman to save her life or health. In clearly hazardous medical situations, the rabbis legislated against even the procreational commandment; she is not to subject herself to physical risk. Once again, the Torah is to be "set aside" when existing life or health is threatened.

With so pro-natalist a general and specific tradition, the Jewish response has been understandably welcoming to new reproductive techniques, such as in-vitro fertilization (IVF). The announcement came from Oldham, England, in 1977, of the successful birth of a healthy baby by bringing sperm and egg together in a Petri dish. This was to overcome the obstacle of blocked Fallopian tubes in the mother, or insufficient sperm motility in the father, or similar impediments. Some faith groups at first demurred: How can one violate natural law or deviate from the natural process, whereby husband and wife, unassisted, see to the conception and gestation of the embryo?

Our response is that the matter need not be affected by concepts of natural law. We do not worship nature or regard its laws as insurmountable. On the contrary, the process of creation is ongoing, and we seek to be "partners with God" in conquering and controlling nature. Hence we applaud efforts to dam the rivers and prevent flooding, to use lightning rods, or even air conditioners, to overcome the tyranny of natural elements. We circumcise infant males, rather than stand back and declare nature perfect. The climax of the Creation narrative in Genesis describes the Sabbath as ordained at a point in Creation when God had, in the literal translation, "ceased from His work which He had created to do." "Created to do"? What does that mean?, the rabbis ask. It means that God created much yet to be done, much for us to do now that we are here on earth, in order to be partners in the continuation of the creative process.

Our "partnership" is a limited one, it must be said before going further. It allows for healing and restoring to wholeness, not to altering that wholeness. Genetic therapy to remove illness or defect is far and distinct from genetic engineering to alter human forms. To address with needed therapy the gene or genes for, say dwarfism, or diabetes, or multiple sclerosis, is to do divine work of restoration to health, this time in the genetic stage just as much as in the somatic stage. Both are expressions of the mandate to heal. This does not "interfere with God's will" anymore than restoring an object lost by its owner, which the Torah bids us to do energetically, or the similar restoration of a patient's lost health by the skill and efforts of the physician. Ethical Monotheism, which is Judaism, means that one God does both the good and the bad, but our ethical mandate, our limited partnership, is only to do the good, such as help the poor and heal the sick. To transgress that boundary and engineer new human forms is not to make whole but to remake, with necessarily subjective and untested blueprints. Genetic therapy has great promise for health; genetic engineering poses great danger for the human image of God.

Cloning is somewhere in between these two pursuits, and also comes in two possibilities. Reproductive cloning, by which a cell of one gender is enucleated and then reproduced in exact duplicates, made vivid in some fictional narratives, is not among the permissible choices. It need only be remembered that the animal Dolly, used as the model for human cloning, was born after 217 defective outcomes, which is bad enough for animals but unthinkable for humans. Even in a successful human production of duplicates, there is the unethical deprivation of a person's individuality, and the creation of the ultimate "identity crisis." On the other hand, therapeutic as opposed to reproductive cloning is the cloning of an organ to serve as a replacement for an ailing one, and thus to restore health to the one in need.

To return to the idea of partnership in our pronatalist efforts, giving nature a little help by circumventing impediments to natural conception through use of the Petri dish is acceptable, even meritorious. Furthermore, we have already "improved upon" nature by the very institution of marriage. Man is not naturally monogamous;

primitives used to mate indiscriminately. Religion and civilization have brought us beyond all this by instituting marriage and known paternity/maternity. Most importantly, a great *mitzvah* is being done here: The desire of a woman for offspring is a deeply human one, and helping her realize this desire, even through recourse to the laboratory but with safeguards against abuse, is a positively human deed. R. David Bleich greeted the news of the birth of Baby Louise by writing, as early as 1978, that we are awaiting more long-term evidence of the health of IVF births, so that this technology "can be a welcome means of bestowing the happiness and fulfillment of parenthood upon otherwise childless couples." Since the phenomenon first greeted us, IVF clinics have multiplied across the country and world, and the current estimate is that about 100,000 babies are here because of *in vitro* assistance. More, the chances for individual success in IVF efforts have greatly improved: The American Fertility Association reports that whereas the success rate in 1998 was 12% of attempts, the rate increased to 25% by the year 2005.

Nor would we be deterred, in our embrace of IVF, by another opposing view, expressed in a socialized-medicine context: "IVF is here to overcome a condition of blocked Fallopian tubes, a result of pelvic inflammation, in turn caused by a syphillitic infection. Like AIDS, this comes from sinful misconduct; we should deny government funding for both." Needless to say, the Jewish medico-moral position roundly rejects this idea. It tells us that we have a mandate to heal, regardless of any supposed etiology of the illness.

Where IVF cannot help overcome obstacles, *in vivo* fertilization may be necessary. Where a woman is capable of ovulation but not of gestation, the ovum is lavaged out and implanted in the womb of another woman. But then the question of maternity is raised: Who is the real mother? In the Talmud's imagery, "there are three partners in the birth of the human child—the father, the mother, and God." The father gives his share, the mother hers, and God gives the soul. Actually, the mother gives more than an equal share, if that can be said. The genetic endowment of the father is matched both by the mother's genetic endowment, the ovum, and her gestational environment and nurture, the womb. If these two contributions are now divided between two women, one supplying the ovum and the other the womb, which one is the mother? Moreover, in the further case of surrogate mothers, who offer both of these contributions to their sponsors, what maternal claim accrues to the sponsor?

Even these ultramodern phenomena have their precedents in Scripture. Rachel and Leah had their own children, but before and in between these births, they "sponsored" children through their handmaidens Bilhah and Zilpah. These handmaidens, as well as Hagar in Abraham's day, were prototypes of surrogate mothers. But they were free of the sociological problems that complicate the picture today. The biblical "surrogates," all in the same home, did not have a change of heart and insist on keeping the babies for themselves. Nor did the sponsors renege because the babies were not up to their expectations; also, there were no financial arrangements. In today's world, safeguards are needed to protect against abuse or unanticipated problems in surrogacy, which then make it a viable alternative where ordinary pregnancy is not possible.

For *in vivo* fertilization, the question of maternity can be resolved in favor of the conceptional mother by arguing that the genetic, as opposed to the gestational, contribution is the dynamic one, providing the all-important genetic code. Also, the donated zygote can be said to be a nascent being, with the identity of the mother already intact. Also, the first mother's role is not replaceable by technology, but the host mother's is; the gestation could conceivably be done in an incubator. On the other hand, maternity can equally be argued for the host mother, that is, the birth mother, on the ground that a transplanted organ becomes an integral part of the body of the recipient, which means that the recipient of an ovarian transplant becomes the mother. Also, the birth mother gives both nurture and gestation to the embryo.

Moreover, as a congressional committee was told in August, 1984, the legal presumption in favor of the birth mother, publicly known to have delivered a baby, "gives the child and society certainty of identification at the time of birth, which is a protection for both mother and child." Nine months of responsible nurture is a far greater "gift" than the surrender of an ovum, entitling the host far more clearly to the acknowledgment of parenthood. Israeli hospitals have, in such cases, actually listed both mothers on the birth certificate. From a halakhic standpoint, both are indeed the child's mother, meaning that the child owes *kibbud em,* "honor thy... mother" to both of them, and, more to the point, must avoid marriage with children of either of them, to preclude unintentional incest. A related question is that of the ethnic-religious identity of the child. If the birth mother is Jewish and the conceptional mother is not, is the child deemed Jewish or not? This query was resolved by most rabbinic authorities in favor of the religion of the birth mother, on the interesting analogy with the laws of conversion. If a woman converts to Judaism during her pregnancy, the child subsequently born has the mother's new status without further ceremony.

Of course, before *in vitro* or *in vivo* was a gleam in anyone's eye, reproductive assistance was found in artificial insemination. In this clinical procedure, the wife is inseminated with her husband's immotile sperm (AIH) or, when a husband was both infertile and impotent, a donor's sperm (AID) was used. Problems connected with the first of these two involve mainly the procurement of the semen, that is, the avoidance of onanism, as well as the possible admixture of the semen of another to increase fertility, which is disallowed. Problems with the second are the initial determination of some rabbinic authorities that the process is adulterous, making the children illegitimate. Others remind us that adultery is a conscious violation of the marriage vows by illicit intimacy, nothing like this clinical procedure. The result is that adultery is not involved and consequent illegitimacy does not happen.

Nonetheless, resort to AID does sever the human, family bond and it does conceal or obscure paternity, an important factor in Jewish law. The children might later unwittingly marry their siblings, unknown paternity having led to the grave sin of incest. Hence, R. Mosheh Feinstein and others had recommended use of a non-Jewish donor to reduce that likelihood. Instances of cancellation of marriage plans, where clinical information identified the donor as related, have already surfaced. Despite apprehensions, however, the procedures can be acceptable where, of course, the natural alternative is unavailable. The fact that the procedure itself is acceptable in the absence of options also means that it is theoretically permissible in the case of an unmarried woman. Yet, the sociological context argues against it. To deliberately give a child one parent instead of two is hardly the ethical path for the welfare of either mother or child.

Does fulfilling the *mitzvah* of *p'ru ur'vu* require resort to IVF in the case of sterility or barrenness? Actually not, because a *mitzvah*, in the sense of an obligation, only obtains when it is normally possible to accomplish it. Before these modern reproductive technologies became available, and before it was knowable whether the impediment was on his side or her side, there are instances in the legal literature in which the question was submitted to the rabbinic authorities. The husband asked whether he needed to divorce his wife and try to marry someone with whom he could sire children. The rabbi would answer that the injunction of *p'ru ur'vu* does not require him to separate from the woman he loves; nor may he ask her to accept a divorce when she was true to her marriage vows in accordance with her abilities. Let him rather look for other *mitzvot* to take the place of this one. He could, for example, study more Torah—or they could adopt a child. True, adoption would not technically constitute *p'ru ur'vu*, because a new life is not brought into being. But it accomplishes an unending *mitzvah* of kindness to a child in need. It gives ongoing foster and nurture to a child over many years—surely a great *mitzvah* in the sense of a good deed.

As stated above, though these Assisted Reproductive Technologies offer relief from barrenness and infertility, they are not to be chosen above relief the natural way. Nor, again, is there a duty to pursue them in order to fulfill the *mitzvah* of *p'ru ur'vu*, above and beyond one's normal efforts. In the hierarchy of alternatives, adoption might seem the far better course, although the apprehension of unknown paternity applies here, too. Hence the identity of natural parents should be made knowable to the child or to a readily accessible friend. From a psychological standpoint, one school of thought prefers adoption to recourse to the above, because this avoids a residual resentment by the husband. That is, if his wife had to receive artificial insemination from another, the child will have the mother's genetic heritage, which is a plus; but the husband is left out entirely, which is a minus. When adoption takes place, neither parent has genetic input, which is a minus; but there is also no resentment or jealousy or reminder of the husband's disproportionate inadequacy, which is a plus.

An additional consideration in all of the above is the matter of lineage, *"yichus"* in its objective sense, which is also an important concept in the Jewish tradition. To know and identify one's ancestors, and to hope to give them immortality by advancing their righteous aspirations, lends another spiritual dimension to one's own life and places it in a larger context of significance. Hence the prevalent custom of naming a child after, say, a grandparent, giving a "second chance" to the ancestor and an inspiration to the descendant. In AIH and *in vitro*, family integrity and lineage remain clear; in the others, it must be sought and affirmed.

Through normal pregnancy and its variations, then, the *mitzvah* and desideratum of natalism can be pursued—but all in keeping with the health and wellbeing of the mother. The principle of *pikkuach nefesh* governs here, too, as we are reminded in a bold and striking statement from none other than *Chatam Sofer*, a pre-eminent rabbinic authority of the nineteenth century. When a question was directed to him about a woman for whom pregnancy would be hazardous (Resp. *Even HaEzer*, 20), his memorable response was, "Childbearing builds the world. But a woman need not build the world by destroying herself."

CHAPTER FIVE

ABORTION AND STEM-CELL RESEARCH

At public hearings on the matter of abortion, I have made the point that the idea of women's rights, or of reproductive freedom, cannot be admissible as an argument in favor of the practice. Nor can we even accept the "right to privacy" as justification thereof, which is the basis for the U.S. Supreme Court's guarantee of access to abortion, as set forth in the famous Roe v. Wade decision of 1973. If abortion is murder, then none of these reasons can be adduced to allow such an act. Just as a mother cannot put to death a grown child on the grounds that he or she is the fruit of her own womb, neither can she do so before birth on the grounds of the right to privacy or of "freedom to do with her body as she sees fit." If abortion is murder, feticide is then as forbidden as homicide, and there are no personal rights of the mother. But if—only if—abortion is not murder, then other considerations, such as the prior concern for the welfare of the mother, even the "right to choose," can come into play.

Abortion is not the same as murder, vociferous claims to the contrary notwithstanding (and a questionably authentic recent responsum notwithstanding). It cannot be murder in Jewish law because murder is one of the three cardinal transgressions which require martyrdom instead. Rather than commit 1) murder of the innocent, 2) public idolatry or apostasy, or 3) gross sexual immorality, such as adultery-incest, one has to surrender his or her own life in martyrdom. All the rest of the Torah is in the category of *ya'avor v'al yehareg*, "let one transgress rather than die"—part of our principle of *pikkuach nefesh*. But not so for murder of the innocent. Hence, if abortion were declared tantamount to murder, a mother would not be allowed to abort her pregnancy even to save her own life, which is obviously not the case.

There is—need it be stated?—no commandment that reads "Thou shalt not kill." It reads "Thou shalt not murder"—*lo tirtzach*, not *lo taharog*. The difference is in the circumstances. Killing is allowed in self-defense, in war, by the sentencing court, even against the prowler in one's home. In these situations, the victim is no longer innocent; he has forfeited his protection under the commandment. He must, of course, do so consciously; he must have deliberately placed himself in a position of attack or of threat in order to lose this statutory protection. Another such category is that of *rodef*, the aggressor, who may also be killed if there is no other way to halt his pursuit or aggression of a third party. The Talmud considers declaring the fetus in a threatening pregnancy to be a *rodef*, an aggressor against its mother, and making that the reason for permitting abortion. But the Talmudic source proceeds to reject that reasoning, suggesting even that the mother herself could be called "the pursuer," by virtue of a physical or anatomical condition that would threaten continuation of the pregnancy. In that case, "perhaps God is the pursuer," says the Talmud, declaring the situation "an act of God."

Now if the fetus is not an aggressor, why else, then, permit abortion? The only valid ground for permitting even therapeutic abortion is that the fetus is not yet a human person. This means that killing admittedly happens here, but not murder. Killing is the taking of the life of, say, an animal or chicken, or of a human who forfeits his immunity by an act of aggression. ("They shoot horses, don't they?" is called a humane thing to do, but not a human thing, as in the case of euthanasia. Humans have the "Image of God" quality and civilization gives them immunity until they forfeit it.) We keep ourselves from the cardinal sin of murder if the victim is either not human or not innocent. The usual question is wrongly asked: When does life begin? The question must rather be: When does life begin to be human? To have discovered a heartbeat in the fetus does not prove it human; it only proves it alive. And the difference between fetal life and human life is not determined by the biologist or the physician or the human court. It is the determination by the religion or the culture that declares when life begins to be human. Of course, this does not make the fetus fair game for destruction—except in a contest between the rights of actual vs. potential life.

At a conference in Rome under the auspices of the Vatican, I pointed out that a life-threatening pregnancy is certainly warrant for abortion. A

Catholic physician rose to challenge my position. She herself had sustained such a pregnancy, she said. Her doctor had counseled abortion, but her priest forbade it. She obeyed her priest, and the child was born without incident. I hesitated to respond to her personal ordeal, but a priest present at that conference did better: "Yes," he said "You, as a Catholic woman, are duty-bound to listen to your priest, who will tell you abortion is wrong. But a Jewish woman is equally duty-bound to listen to her rabbi, who will tell her that Jewish law forbids her to put her life in danger, even if the danger turns out to be a false alarm." I was delighted that that priest was properly informed, and would articulate so well the principle of *pikkuach nefesh*, a basic theme of the present book.

Another such clarifying confrontation took place at a lecture back home in New York City, when a Catholic listener rose to question. She began: "Don't you believe in the Bible?" "Oh yes," I replied. "Well, the Bible says 'Therefore, choose life.' Since abortion is the taking of life, how can you allow it?" "Because," I answered, "when *you* see the words 'choose life' in the Bible, and when *we* see them, we're seeing different things. From a Catholic viewpoint, essentially otherworldly in orientation, you see 'life' as life in the next world. Otherwise, why would you allow the demise of the mother? Yet, you feel that the mother, already baptized as an infant, will indeed be choosing life for herself in the next world. But when *we* look at those words, we think of life in this world, and so we strive to save the mother, to save an existing life." "And how do I know this?," I continued. "Because the Talmud, in support of its principle of *pikkuach nefesh*, tells us: 'Violate [for the patient] this Sabbath, so he will be here to keep many Sabbaths.' In other words, we want to choose life here on earth, to 'stick around,' so to speak, and a therapeutic abortion is therefore indicated, even mandated."

Illustrative of the difference, albeit technical, between murder and killing is the following report: Rabbi Issar Unterman, a chief rabbi of Israel who died in 1965, was firmly opposed to abortion, which he called "akin to murder." In his legal writings, he describes an episode in Lithuania during the First World War, where a Jewish doctor was ordered by a soldier to terminate the pregnancy of his woman companion. When the doctor refused on grounds of conscience, the soldier drew his weapon and repeated the order at gunpoint. Rabbi Unterman writes: Though I oppose abortion, had I been there to be asked, I would, in those circumstances, have forbidden the doctor to martyr himself. Feticide just cannot be made equal to homicide, and the doctor must act accordingly.

Less dramatic, but instructive nonetheless, is the response of the *Gaon* of Rogatchev in the previous century. When a husband pointed to an abortion by his wife as grounds for his intended divorce, as murder might be, the *Gaon*, Rabbi Joseph Rosin, rejected the claim. You might use the term rhetorically, was his ruling, but literal murder it's not.

In a previous book, *Birth Control in Jewish Law,* I have set forth aspects of the legal parameters of the larger abortion question, so they will not be repeated here. The reader can consult pages 251 to 294 and pages 338 to 347 of that book on matters such as *ubar yerekh immo,* of any "juridical personality" the fetus may have, the law of homicide in the Torah, the law of accidental feticide in Exodus, the rabbinic understanding and the Septuagint version thereof, the consequences for the Christian and the Noahide positions, the issue of "ensoulment," as well as the bearing of such concepts as "original sin" on the question. I traced a stricter and more lenient strand in practical rulings, associated with Maimonides on the former and Rashi on the latter. But the pivotal Mishnah does deserve to be repeated here. It states:

> If a woman has [life-threatening] difficulty in childbirth, one dismembers the fetus within her, [even] limb by limb, because her life takes precedence over its life.

> Once its head (or its "greater part") has emerged, it may not be touched, because we do not set aside one life for another.

Aside from the other implications of this Mishnah, its first half makes clear that actual life takes precedence over potential life and, in doing so, it sets aright some misleading slogans of our day.

The "right to life" assertion more correctly belongs to the classic Jewish position, and is a phrase wrongly applied to the anti-abortion stance. Also, its opposite, the "pro-choice" position is a misnomer, because the right of "choice" is irrelevant, *pikkuach nefesh* insisting that the woman has no choice when her life is in danger. "Right to life" is not applicable to the abortion question at all; abortion is really a matter of "right to be born." A right to be born is not absolute; it is relative to the welfare of the mother. The right to be born is hardly different from the right to be conceived.

But just as the Mishnah makes the fetus secondary to the mother before birth, so it rejects any such distinction after birth. The second half of this brief but pregnant Mishnah negates another popular slogan, that of the "quality of life." By teaching that the newborn baby "may not be touched" because it already is a *nefesh*, a human being, it is saying that its life is as inviolate as that of its mother. Its right to life is then absolute. If quality of life were the determining factor in who shall live, it would be absurd to see the newborn as equal in claim to that of its mother. The mother has her achievements and social connectedness, her proven viability. The infant has none of these yet, is not even considered *bar kayyama*, viable, for another 30 days. Still, we reject any notion of relative quality; the operative motto is rather "sanctity of life" for all who possess human life. From the moment of its birth, the life of the newborn is sacred, as indivisibly and inalienably sacred as that of its mother. Again, this is where true right to life obtains, for while a right to be born is relative to the welfare of the mother, right to life is not relative to the mother's or anyone's welfare. It means no person has to apologize for living, neither to parents, to physicians, to society, or to self. It also means, hopefully, that society, through its institutions, will help or spare the parents in attending to the needs of its handicapped.

The current issue of embryonic stem cell research bids us to come back for a deeper look at the question of "when does life begin to be human?" If we have determined that the fetus is potential life, what do we say about the pre-fetal embryo? The embryo in its earlier stage is a blastocyst, a cluster of undifferentiated cells which, if fertilized *in vitro*, has not yet been implanted in the uterus, not yet on its way to become a fetus. At this stage the blastocyst could give rise to the specialized cells of various body tissues, including heart, kidney, and brain cells, and could, in theory, be used to replace cells that have become defective in people with disease or disability. Scientists promise great therapeutic benefit from the results of research on the cells of these embryos, that they may hold the key to developing medicines and therapies for a variety of diseases and conditions, including Alzheimer's, Parkinson's, diabetes, and spinal cord injuries, indeed improvements in about 70 diseases for which the research shows promise.

On the other hand, "somatic" cells from born individuals or adults, taken, say, from the umbilical cord, or from the heart cells or brain marrow, can also help, but these adult cells are called multipotent, as opposed to totipotent, or at least pluripotent, the latter describing the embryonic variety. These can do "everything," and are the subject of both the medical excitement and the theological controversy of the day.

In the scientific community, the therapeutic possibilities that can result from this research are enormous. Though there is little evidence so far of successful human application, there seems to be no dissent about the reality of such possibilities. Also, there is little dissent about the number of people who stand to benefit greatly. Steven L. Stice, a prominent stem-cell researcher at the University of Georgia, says estimates indicate that there are 128 million people who suffer from a disease that could be cured or treated with stem cells. On the other hand, James Thomson of the University of Wisconsin played down the dramatic possibilities of curing disease by transplanting stem cells, but will fight for the research because of the therapeutic science it will yield sooner.

Of the diseases for which relief is most promising, one of them is Parkinson's, the affliction suffered by the popular actor, Michael J. Fox. As he withdrew from his successful acting career, he wrote a persuasive Op-Ed piece for the New York Times, where he asked that the opponents of embryonic stem-cell research "explain to those of us with debilitating disease—indeed, to all of us— why it is more pro-life to throw away stem cells than to put them to work saving lives."

But the Catholic Church and some conservative Protestant groups insist that human life already exists in embryos, and the taking of that life is not justified even for its therapeutic probabilities. Arguably, the Catholic position has moved historically from seeing potential human life—as had been the case—to seeing actual human life in unimplanted embryos. But the latter, more extreme view, is the more determinative one in today's political reality. A group of conservative lawmakers, headed by Sen. Sam Brownback of Kansas, has vowed to block any move by the National Institutes of Health that would advocate liberalizing the use of federal funds for embryonic stem-cell research. President George W. Bush reached a compromise at the beginning of his first term, in August, 2001, restricting research to existing "lines" of cells but prohibiting the creation of new ones. Although the compromise was politically necessary, and perhaps from his standpoint even morally necessary, advocates see it as wholly inadequate for the needs of planned research.

It is likewise important to point out that opposition to use of discarded embryos is based on the fear of what it might lead to. The apprehension is that such could lead to the creation of embryos for the purpose of being discarded, so that they can be used for desirable research. The argument is reminiscent of what transpired a generation earlier in the matter of fetal tissue. There was much discussion about the possible use of fetal tissue, from aborted fetuses, to be implanted in the brain areas of adult victims of Parkinson's or Alzheimer's in order to improve secretion of neurotransmitter substances, relieving their symptoms significantly. This procedure entails less rejection because the basic HLA tissue type is not expressed until 12 weeks of fetal life. In a famous news item, a young, unmarried woman offered to receive artificial insemination, to gestate and then abort, so as to make fetal tissue available for her afflicted father. The father publicly disavowed the intended procedure, regarding it as ethically unacceptable. On a national level, the research with fetal tissue was banned, under the auspices of President Ronald Reagan, because the apprehension was there, too, that this would lead to increased abortion. When, sadly, ex-President Reagan himself became an Alzheimer's patient, some were heard to say that advances in fetal tissue research, had the research been allowed to continue, might ironically have been of great help to him. In reply, his wife Nancy declared that he was principled in his belief, and would not have changed his policy even if he could have foreseen a benefit to himself.

Rabbinic opinion is virtually unanimous that human status cannot be ascribed to pre-implantation embryos. Though fertilized, they are yet to be implanted in the womb, where the process may or may not succeed. A fetus, as precious as it is, is only potential in its status, as compared with a born child's actual human status. But the earlier embryo has even less; it has only the pre-potential status of individual zygotes, of sperm and ovum. They, too, are to be protected and treasured—but where they failed to impregnate they ought certainly to be used for healing. To discard them is wrong, although that happens routinely in IVF clinics when implantation was unsuccessful. To avoid using them because such might encourage creation of embryos expressly for this purpose, or lead to intentional non-implantation of available ones, is likewise wrong. These failed embryos are outside the womb and are microscopic clumps of undifferentiated cells; they are destined to be destroyed and thus to end any potential for life or healing.

The principle of *pikkuach nefesh*, yes, a basic theme of this book, steps forward again to point the way in this matter. Once the determination is clear that human life is not destroyed by the use of embryonic stem cells, then their vast therapeutic potential demands that they be used for healing and relief—demands that they become instruments of *pikkuach nefesh* for the health and wellbeing of humanity. We fervently hope that the policy in Washington will join that of Israel, where unfettered progress is being pursued in this area, as well as the ongoing efforts in Australia and England.* As of this writing, there is heightened activ-

---

* South Korean scientists have recently announced taking stem cells from cloned human embryos, which would suffer

ity on both sides of the issue, with advocates of embryonic stem cell exploration becoming more vocal, and with Congress actually passing legislation in defiance of the White House to provide federal funds for it. Regardless of these political and philosophic challenges to his view on the matter, President Bush promises to veto the new legislation.

Meanwhile, research activity is blossoming in individual states in the U.S., beginning with New Jersey and continuing elsewhere—but most ambitiously in California, where Proposition 76 approved the expenditure of three billion dollars over the next ten years for this specific purpose. Properly, medical ethicists are beginning to write the rules to keep the program and the spending on target. Oversight committees will be established to approve and monitor the research. California will become the front-runner in the field, most likely inviting Israeli scientists to share what they have learned in their head-start in study and with their dedication in attitude.

Israel's dedication has already led to the creation there of a consortium of several companies involved in cutting-edge laboratory work in the field, which makes regular progress reports. Despite its small numbers vis-à-vis the larger countries, Israel is disproportionately represented in all

---

less rejection in the healing of the source body. The cloning itself, however, has aroused greater fear and opposition here.

the natural sciences and, motivated by its values, is forging ahead. With or without White House policy change, the consortium looks forward to gaining U.S. Food and Drug Agency approval for the embryonic stem cells it creates for therapy, for *pikkuach nefesh*.

CHAPTER SIX

ORGAN
TRANSPLANTATION

The matter of organ donations—cadaver organs, that is, as opposed to organs from live donors—has its theoretic beginnings in the matter of autopsies. Here, a competing principle is in conflict with our subject one, and the resolution of the conflict is interesting and significant

Our subject principle is *pikkuach nefesh*, the *mitzvah* of saving a life, a fundamental consideration that takes precedence over almost all other options. The challenger here is *k'vod ha-met*, of treating the deceased with the respect due a body that so recently housed the soul and that still represents a person in his or her individuality. This latter principle is usually expressed in its negative form, namely the prohibition of *nivvul ha-met*, desecration of the dead. This would rule out post-mortem autopsies for information that does not directly serve the purpose of saving life.

The halakhic narrative has its resolution, or its major turning point, in a historic ruling by R. Yechezkel Landau, known as *Noda Biyhudah*, of eighteenth-century Prague. The rabbi was in receipt of a written query from a physician in London who had lost a patient to "stones," gallstones or kidney stones. He felt that if he could set aside consideration of *nivvul ha-met* in order to autopsy his patient, he might learn more about the cause and nature of the disease and perhaps save the life of the next patient similarly afflicted.

R. Landau's responsum was the anticipated balancing of the two principles. After all, obtaining greater knowledge through post-mortem autopsy could make it easier to save life in the future. But it's not fair to the deceased to mutilate this body in the uncertain hope of helping another, of possibly acquiring enough specific information that could justify setting aside the inhibition against mutilating the deceased. True, saving a life is paramount, but we need more probability that it will indeed ensue, and we need a more evident connection between the autopsy and its life-saving benefit.

A phrase of just two words used by R. Landau in his responsum to this question resonated through the decades and through the situations of need. The words are *"choleh l'faneinu,* the patient before us," meaning that whereas an autopsy cannot be permitted in the hope that it might contribute to general medical knowledge somewhere sometime, it indeed could if there is a "patient before us" who can benefit, thus activating the principle of direct and timely *pikkuach nefesh*. After all, this latter principle could only permit, to further illustrate, the violation of the Sabbath for the emergent act of healing, but not to prepare on the Sabbath the healing for a possible case thereafter.

So our formula was now available to balance the two imperatives, and it received significant

: 81

amplification in later years. R. Chayyim Ozer
Grodzinsky, for example, was no stranger to the
technology of the 1940's in Poland, where it is said
he would respond to queries in Jewish law by
speaking on two telephones at the same time. It
was clear to him that a patient can be anywhere in
the world, transformed as our world is into a
global village by the fact of instantaneous com-
munication, and qualify as a "patient before us."
So if someone in need in Vienna can be helped by
information emerging in Jerusalem or London or
New York, an autopsy for that purpose ought to
be done.

It follows, then, that removal of an organ from
a cadaver that can save the life of the recipient-in-
waiting is similar—a similar mandate to save existing life even by desecrating the body of the deceased. Yet, even if the logic was clear, there has
remained strong inhibition against cadaver transplantation. Why?

One reason is the sense that the body should
remain intact. This follows from the requirement
that proper burial be provided for the body and
all its parts. In the case of amputation, by surgery
or by accident, the severed limbs must be given
proper burial, even if not together with the body
from which they came. This is *k'vod ha-met*, the respect that we owe to the body. Some feel that the
promise of *t'hiyyat ha-metim*, of physical resurrection of the body in Messianic times, requires that
the body await this miracle in intact form.

Spiritual immortality, the permanence of the soul after its liberation from the body, is the more natural prospect, according to Maimonides. But the miracle of physical resurrection is also promised. As a miracle, then, it can come about even with a decomposed body. Medieval Jewish philosophers, beginning with Saadia Gaon, used to be taunted by skeptics of *t'hiyyat ha-metim*. What happens, they would ask, if a person is devoured by a lion, and then the lion is consumed in a forest fire—what happens then to resurrection? The answer, of course, is that resurrection is a miracle. Just as God can perform the miracle after the body has been decomposed with the passage of time, so can He do so with a body no longer intact for other reasons.

And, hard as it is to contemplate that our bodies soon decompose and that we are left with bones and skeleton only, this is obviously the case. In the book of Exodus, at the high point of the drama of escape from Egyptian bondage, Moses reminds the people of the pledge made to Joseph, that they would bring him along when they left Egypt. The text does not say that they had pledged to bring his body with them, but "his bones." They kept their pledge and brought along "*atzmot Yosef*, the bones of Joseph," to the Promised Land.

If the permanence of the soul after its liberation from the body is the more natural prospect, Maimonides and the others accepted the idea of physical resurrection, too, because it was a doctrine. Physical revival would take place to fulfill the promised miracle, but would be of short duration, giving way to lasting spiritual presence, in keeping with the nature of the soul vs. that of the body. In a purely this-worldly and halakhic context, then, the saving of another life here and now is the first consideration.

This is not to say that concern for the intactness of the body was the primary reason for antipathy to cadaver organ transplantation. R. Mosheh Feinstein, who clearly permitted it to save the life of the donee, stipulated that the permission of the family be first obtained. But clearly the family has no ownership of the body, and their consent cannot be an issue. Yet, this sage sensed the anguish a family could feel knowing that the body of their loved one was subjected to this procedure. Obtaining permission would help in placating and reassuring them. Another aspect of the legal protection of the cadaver is the prohibition against deriving financial benefit therefrom. Knowing this fact would thwart grave-robbing and other exploitation of the defenseless deceased. But here, too, transfer of the body part to a living recipient, to be itself revived, for the *mitzvah* of saving life, overcomes that consideration.

Yet, none of this prevented the issue from being a matter of prolonged contention, with protests by some *charedim* in Jerusalem against Hadassah Hospital, for example, for its practice of autopsies. After much contention, a concordat was entered into in 1954 between Chief Rabbi Isaac

Herzog and Hadassah Hospital, which limited the performance of post-mortems to the following circumstances: a) where life could be saved by direct medical application of information garnered therefrom, b) where life could be saved forensically, namely by acquitting a defendant in proving that death was not caused by his actions, and c) where lives in the family could be saved when the condition was demonstrably hereditary.

The direct connectedness between the taking of data, or of organs, by autopsy and between its life-saving use, accordingly, excludes use of organ banks. Halakhically-sanctioned organ-donation cards, for attachment to drivers' licenses or the like, must state that organs are not available for storage or accumulation, but only for immediate transplantation. Since most vital organs are already in pressing demand, this caution is almost unnecessary. In one instructive case, the balance in the legal provision has recently been adjusted: The rule had been that human skin should not be stored against possible need but acquired at time of need. An incident in the Israeli army, wherein troops were injured by "friendly fire," changed all that. The incident created the need for quick skin transplants to heal the damage from severe burns. But the nearest available skin for the purpose was in Holland, and the hours that passed awaiting its transport allowed the condition to worsen. The rabbis concluded that since there is clearly a time factor, they would now permit the storage of human skin so that it be accessible without deleterious delay.

None of these strictures apply to organ donations from living persons, but other considerations do. Before liver transplants were possible with only part of the organ—that is, when the operation required the sacrificial donation of an entire liver—that donation would be forbidden on the grounds of suicide, since one is not ordinarily permitted to give his life to save another's. But to donate part of the liver now is like what it was to donate one kidney. Since the latter does put the donor at some risk, there is no obligation to do so, only permission. The surgery involved, and the effect on the donor's longevity, are reasons for declining to do so; but with proper medical counsel, the donor is still permitted this act of supreme kindness. Bone marrow transplants carry much less risk, and their donation is much closer to an obligation. Blood donations are clearly closest to a risk-free *mitzvah*.

Returning to transplantation from a cadaver, a significant step forward in principle and in practice was advocated by Chief Rabbi Issar Unterman, who included corneal transplants among the reasons justifying desecration of the deceased. Restoring the donee's sight may not actually save his life, but saving his sight is virtually equal in human gain. Also, a person's life can literally be saved, in such circumstances as crossing the street, by his ability to see what threatens him.

More than 84,000 Americans are waiting for donated organs to replace their diseased ones. In Israel, it is estimated that more than 100 people die each year waiting for organs. The issue and the opportunities came to the fore in 1995, when Alisa Flatow was murdered by terrorists. Her father, Stephen Flatow, rushed to Israel to her side and communicated by telephone with R. Mosheh Tendler, back in the United States, who advised him to allow the organ donations to take place. As many as five lives were saved by that decisive act of kindness. Rabbi Tendler later noted that a deceased person can potentially save nine lives—by offering two kidneys, two separate halves of the liver, two lungs, two corneas, and yes, a heart.

But for the heart, we must pause. In transplants from the deceased, the one gift that is the subject of ample debate and caution is that of the heart. The liver, too, requires the donor to be at least brain-dead, but even if the heart has also stopped beating, the liver remains transplantable. While the other organs are taken only after death is definite according to most criteria, the heart would be useless to the donee if we were to wait for full cardiac death. Taking the heart without waiting might mean hastening the death of the donor, which is clearly forbidden, in order to help the donee. For heart transplants, then, we first need the chapter on the determination of death.

CHAPTER SEVEN

DETERMINATION OF DEATH

Criteria for the determination of death appear in the Talmud almost incidentally, in a purely practical context. The subject there (*Yoma* 82a, 85a) is something else entirely, i.e. guidance on saving a life in the face of Sabbath prohibitions. That unlikely context happens to be a source-text for the concept, and then the principle, of our present theme, that of *pikkuach nefesh* for all its cases.

But determination of death does issue from the same discussion. We are instructed: If one chances upon a collapsed building on the Sabbath, he should proceed with what is an apparent violation thereof. He should remove enough of the debris to ascertain whether a victim of the collapse can still be saved. Having found a victim, he should begin clearing debris from the rest of the victim's body, starting from the top and going downward. "Examine him at the nostrils," is the first directive of the Talmud. "Examine him at the heart," is its second directive. Once breath in the nostrils, or pulsation in the heart, can be detected, that's enough to continue violating the Sabbath, to quickly remove the person from under the debris, or give him or her life-saving treatment. The implication is that if nothing can be detected at the nostrils or at the heart—no cardiopulmonary activity, that is—then there is no chance of saving a life, and therefore no justification for further labors otherwise forbidden. (The Talmud goes on to caution that there may be other victims buried more deeply under the debris, who may still be hanging onto life. These should not be neglected because of what was found with the first ones.)

The basic cardiopulmonary criteria, then, are historically the standard for declaration of death and all the implications thereof, and have been firmly held through the centuries. After Maimonides' Code and the *Shulchan Arukh,* R. Moses Sofer, the *Chatam Sofer* of nineteenth-century Hungary, gave a systematic treatment of the subject. He added the stipulation of Rashi that the patient be motionless, to preclude the possibility of declaring one dead who satisfied these criteria but who manifested other signs of activity. But anything like brain death, a so-called neurological determination of death, would have been clearly excluded by his affirmation of the halakhic guidelines as set forth in the Talmud. *Chatam Sofer,* it should be noted, also advised against being too strict in the observance of these criteria, because the extra caution might cause a delay in the burial of a clearly deceased person. That would incur a violation of *halanat ha-met,* of desecration of the dead by postponing proper burial.

*Chatam Sofer'*s long disquisition on the subject, as it happens, was occasioned by an event that troubled him, one that involved Moses Mendelssohn and a government order. In 1772, the Duke of Mecklenburg had decreed that the deceased not be interred until 3 days after death, to avoid any mistake, and Mendelssohn sought to please him by showing that this, too, could be consistent with Jewish law.

His contemporary, R. Yaakov Emden, argued strongly against the Duke's decree and insisted on immediate burial to prevent *halanat ha-met*. When the debate arose again in the days of *Chatam Sofer*, he took up the cudgels and militated against the position of Mendelssohn, as *Chatam Sofer* generally did against leaders of the *Haskalah* (Enlightenment) or of Reform. In the process he gave us the comprehensive statement in a responsum (*Yoreh Deah* 338), referred to above, on death and its determination, in theory and in practice.

The twentieth century brought a wholly new challenge to the adequacy of the historic criteria, now that heart transplantation became a welcome possibility. After the pioneering successes of Dr. Christian Bernard in South Africa and Dr. Michael DeBakey in Texas, the halakhic question was put to R. Mosheh Feinstein, the acknowledged authority and decisor of the age. His response was clearly negative, that because the heart was taken before the donor was really dead—since the heart was necessarily still beating—and since the donee's life could be shortened by a less than successful procedure, the surgeons are guilty of double murder!

As time went on, it was easier to argue against the second half than the first. The threat to the recipient abated significantly with the progress of medical training, skill, and experience, and as the official success rate registered an undeniable gain. Against this background, R. Feinstein's distinguished son-in-law, R. Mosheh Tendler, wrote in support of heart transplantation as an expression of the basic life-saving *mitzvah*. Other rabbis took him to task, demanding that he explain why he is presuming to negate the responsum of none other than his illustrious and ultimately authoritative father-in-law who wrote so clearly in opposition. His answer was to point to the date of R. Feinstein's responsum, namely decades earlier, and call attention to the remarkable progress in the interim for the success rate for the donee. Sardonically, he clinched his argument by saying that his conclusion is now endorsed by none other than Blue Cross Health Insurance. Blue Cross, he said, would not reimburse patients for any procedure that is merely experimental. The fact that this insurer and others now pay the bill is proof that the procedure has graduated from the experimental to the acknowledged, and the benefit to the patient is undisputed. In addition, cyclosporin is now available to neutralize the body's natural rejection of foreign elements, in this case the implanted heart. Cyclosporin, unheard of when R. Feinstein originally wrote on the subject, now immeasurably improves the success rate of all transplant therapy.

The other half of the double-murder charge, that taking a heart from a donor who is dead only neurologically causes his death, remains infinitely harder to disprove. But R. Tendler has made a valiant effort to do so, and his name is famously associated with the affirmative position on brain death as a halakhic criterion. R. David Bleich, also a senior member of the faculty of Yeshiva University, is equally well known for his resistance to the idea, and has written books and articles to that effect.

In the absence of the neurological criterion in the Talmud, the current argument for brain-death acceptance considered, in a new analysis, the respective roles of brain and heart-lungs. The role of the brain was determined to be that of captain, the head, while the other organs were lieutenants following orders. The heart beats and the lungs expand and contract only on orders from the brain. When the brain ceases to initiate orders, the continuing heartbeat and lung activity are only residual, habitual, reflexive, and not sustainable on their own. Reference is also made to the Talmudic mention of the *z'nav ha-l'ta'ah*, the lizard's tail which, after the lizard had been decapitated, continued to convulse. That convulsiveness was clearly not in obedience to the lizard's head after it was severed, but was obviously residual, reflexive, or electric. Brain death is the physiological analog to anatomic decapitation. Decapitation is elsewhere presumed to be synonymous with death, as in the Talmud's rhetorical question, *"p'sik reishei, v'lo yamut?* — can you cut off its head and it won't die?" (This is the Talmud's phrase for assigning responsibility to the doer for the consequences of his actions, inevitable even if unintended.)

Rabbi Dr. Avraham Steinberg of Shaarei Tzedek Hospital in Jerusalem, who made a presentation before the Chief Rabbinate in favor of brain death as actual death, put it this way: Every organ of the body can be resuscitated if it fails. The heart can be revived, lung activity can be coaxed to resume, and the same for liver, kidneys, and so on. But with the brain, once there is lysis (i.e. liquefaction) of the brain cells, there is no way back. The brain, he maintained, is the only organ that, once it dies, the organism itself dies. Nothing is as irreversibly dead for the organism as its brain. It can also be said, though this does not appear in the halakhic arguments, that late-medieval texts in our Prayer Book assume a more determinative role for the brain. There is, for example, the *kavvanah*, the intention-focusing declaration recited before donning the daily *tefillin*, the so-called phylacteries worn on hand and head during morning prayers on weekdays. The part adorning the hand is to dedicate one's actions to God's purposes; the one on the head is to similarly dedicate one's thoughts and aspirations, which latter are here collectively referred to as *"ha-n'shamah she-b'mochi,"* the "soul in my brain."

A high point in the history of the brain-death discussion came with the publication of Harvard Medical School's Ad Hoc Committee on the subject, which defined the condition as unresponsiveness to painful stimuli, and a flat electroencephalogram, reconfirmed after a 24-hour wait. Later versions by the Harvard Committee and by other professional bodies enhanced the quoted requirements, and even included confirmatory blood flow tests, or an apnea test. It was generally specified that the phrase "brain death" should always mean "brain-stem death," that the lower brain, the cerebellum, must have ended its function, not just the cerebrum. Comatose and vegetative conditions result when only the cerebrum dies, but full death comes with cessation of

life in the cerebellum. R. Bleich would hold out for
the dysfunction of the hypothalamus as well.

That the matter remains in dispute is illustrated
in the following consequences: The State of New Jersey has agreed to enact a rare religious-exemption
clause. It empowers individuals, such as caretakers
of those Jewish patients who would not accept brain
death, to refuse to have them declared dead by physicians who do accept it. Rabbis who participate in
this exemption arrangement are aware of the ensu-
ing ethical dilemma. It would mean asking a hospital staff to continue giving treatment to a patient it
regards as deceased. Hence the family of this patient
would seek alternative ways to care for the patient
in and away from the medical facility, consistent
with practical considerations. Duly appreciative of
New Jersey's democratic largesse, the rabbis will not
want to effectively disdain the convictions of a hospital and its staff.

On the other hand, the action of the State of Israel
is remarkable. As mentioned above, Dr. Steinberg of
Shaarei Tzedek Hospital, alongside other learned advocates, made presentations before the Chief Rabbinate on the matter of the acceptability of brain-
death determination. After listening and deliberat-
ing for some time, the rabbis issued their verdict:
Even if the halakhic and scientific arguments in favor of brain death are not absolute, we may be
wrong in hesitating. The *mitzvah* of saving a life is so
great, and the potential of saving many lives is so
clear, that we will hold our theoretical doubts in
abeyance. We will yield to the probability that the

truth may be in favor of permitting heart transplantation—just so that, in the real world, the *mitzvah* of *pikkuach nefesh* can be fulfilled on behalf of those needy patients! Accordingly, in a ruling promulgated in 1986, the Chief Rabbinate permitted the taking of a donor's heart when 1) the etiology of brain damage is known, 2) natural breathing has completely ceased, 3) the brain stem is determined to be destroyed, proven by objective tests such as BAER (brainstem auditory-evoked responses), and 4) these last two elements have persisted for at least 12 hours, in spite of continued intensive care.

The legacy of the late R. Shlomoh Zalman Auerbach of Jerusalem, first-rank decisor on such matters, remains opposed to generalized human heart transplantation, allowing for some specific exceptions. He is an example of sages, giants of halakhic wisdom, who continue in their theoretic cautiousness. They are equally concerned for the imperative of *pikkuach nefesh* but, compelling as that might be, give primacy to the greater fear that existing life might be foreshortened. The functioning Chief Rabbinate, on the other hand, has taken an empirical stand in favor of the procedure and points to abundant theoretic support for confidence that the donor's life is not sacrificed. This does demonstrate the courageous compassion of these rabbinic authorities, and, once again, points to the majestic preeminence of the *mitzvah* to save life and health.

CHAPTER EIGHT

"WHOSE LIFE IS IT?"

J ust as the Talmud offers guidelines for examining whether a victim in a collapsed building might still be alive, thus formulating the parameters of *pikkuach nefesh* to save such victim in spite of the Sabbath, so does it provide directives for a related concern—for attention to one who has clearly died. Its point is that death not be hastened even imperceptibly in following the standard procedure. In that procedure, we must close the eyes of the deceased and bring together the hands and the feet. However, the passage admonishes, if we were to carry out any of these or other requirements a moment too early, while life is still ebbing, we would be guilty of accelerating the death. For, we are told, the soul is likened to the flame on a candle, and to touch a flickering candle is to put out the flame prematurely.

Treatment of the moribund patient, called a *goses*, informs much of the protocol of treatment of the dying. A *goses* may not be touched, for the above reason, unless the touching or moving is to save the life, not inadvertently hurry along its end.

Hastening death can happen by psychological means, not just physical. This apprehension extends to the matter of the deathbed confessional and its wording. We are instructed that a confessional must be couched in the conditional, not the declarative, mode. As cited in Chapter 3 above, one should avoid words which seem to surrender one's will-to-live, such as: "God, I am about to die. May my sins be forgiven, and may I be granted a share in the World to Come." One should instead say "I pray for continued life. If this is not to be, then may my sins be forgiven, etc." We are to forestall the subtle power of suggestion in this manner, and we must certainly stay clear of more obvious self-fulfilling prophecies. This also means that the patient needs to be protected from being informed, unnecessarily, of a distressing diagnosis, considering that the emotional impact of such knowledge can weaken his or her will to live.

The physical hastening of death, especially for reasons of pain or diminished quality of life, is the more obvious apprehension. The issue was captured in terms of "Whose Life Is It, Anyway?," to quote the title of literary and theatrical dramatizations. From the perspective of Judaism, the answer is—not the one implied by the rhetorical "anyway." If "anyway" is deleted, and the question is asked innocently, the answer, to begin with, is that life is not the patient's. It's not his or her life to take, because suicide is as forbidden as is homicide of someone else. Hence, a deed which brings about death, or merely accelerates it unduly, actively or passively, is rejected in principle.

Whose life is it? If life is not the questioner's, is it then for one's family to determine what to do? No, neither is life the family's to take, because members of the family are naturally prejudiced, either in favor or against. Either they care too much for the patient and want the doctors to "try everything," actually to prolong the dying rather than the living, something also to be avoided; or they would hasten death out of genuine, altruistic compassion for the loved one. Conversely, the family could care too little for the patient, consciously or unconsciously, and care too much for ulterior considerations—material, emotional, or otherwise. Prof. Yale Kamisar wrote recently, and counterintuitively, in the Los Angeles Daily [Law] Journal, that "the family should be the last to be asked." Members of the family may seem to be objective, but how can they really be? He points to the husband tending his cancerous wife who, in desperation, appeals to the doctor to "put her out of her misery." What he is often really saying, subconsciously, is "It's time to get on with my own life." Others would understand his words, "Let's put her out of her misery," as meaning possibly, again without conscious awareness, "Let's put her out of *my* misery."

Nor is life the doctor's to take, from the Jewish and indeed from a cross-cultural standpoint. The doctor's mandate is to heal and relieve, not to kill for whatever reason. *Halakhah* yields to the physician's judgment only when he or she offers an opinion that is medical, not personal. It accepts a medical opinion offered about the state of a patient's health or risks for life or death, but never a personal opinion about whether that life, of diminished quality, is worth saving. In fact, because of the doctor's mandate to heal, even most advocates of euthanasia have opposed the idea of physician-assisted suicide. This would violate the physician-patient relationship of trust, as well as that mandate to heal. The trust relationship is, in fact, a problem: The New York State Task Force on Law and Life raises the possibility that this trust might lull us into accepting an assisted suicide from someone whose authoritarian or paternalistic view we might accept implicitly.

Similarly, for reasons of preserving the healing function of medicine, the American Medical Association has declined to allow its members to administer lethal injections in criminal executions. And for the rest of us, the recent series of assisted suicides by Dr. Jack Kevorkian illustrates the difference between his course of action and that of respectable physicians. In the case of his first client, Janet Adkins, it is clear that she only feared possible, future pain; moreover, he took no time to acquaint himself with her real situation, her diagnosis, or her prognosis. As to his later clients, none of them even pointed to physical pain as the reason they sought his help.

Whose life is it, then? Not the patient's, not the family's, not the doctor's. Life is God's, or, stated in different terms, life belongs to the principle that the right to life is inalienable, that it is a gift from the Creator, that it would be blasphemous to cast that gift back ungratefully, and that we, being creatures rather than Creator, are not the arbiters of the end of life for ourselves or fellow humans. And we are creatures "in the image of God," which gives life a sanctity beyond our own estimations thereof, and beyond our right to dispense with.

From vintage dramatic productions like "Whose Life Is It, Anyway?," we zoom ahead to the real-life drama of Terri Schiavo, which was unfolding as I wrote these lines. She was the young victim of brain damage, being fed by tube in a Florida hospital, where the battle raged between her husband, who wanted the tube removed so that she could die, and her parents, who wanted the feeding by tube to continue. The governor, Congress, judges, and the White House had entered the fray, and the issue was fought over whose wishes should prevail, those of husband or those of parents. Yet, the halakhic point of view reminds us of the obvious, that the wishes of neither spouse nor parents—not even of the patient herself—are determinative. This, of course, is not the whole story in the secular or the government's point of view, as was evident in the Nancy Cruzan case of a few years back. There, and in similar cases, the courts needed nothing more than evidence that the patient had expressed her wishes before becoming incapable of doing so.

But if life does not belong to the patient, but to the principle that life is inviolate, then the wishes expressed by—much less inferred from the words of—the patient are insufficient to allow the curtailing of that life. Other members of the family have no more authority to do so, regardless of how close or remote the relationship, before we even consider the stance of Yale Kamisar, above. That stance holds that the family is the *last* to ask because their love for the patient, or the effect of the patient's life or death directly on them, makes them invalid witnesses. Only the unbiased medical opinion of diagnosis and prognosis is admissible here. And even then, any intervention has to be objectively in keeping with what is allowable. Since Michael Schiavo could have been convicted for murder if he put his wife to death in any of the ordinary ways, the "sanctity of marriage" notwithstanding, then what we need to know here is whether removing the tube is murder or not—not who is the one asking for it.

The idea that "the family is the last to ask" shares a halakhic approach, as can be seen from a different corner of the law. There is a famous story in the Talmud (*K'tubot* 104a) where the action of the housemaid of R. Judah Ha-Nasi is described. She so sympathized with his suffering at his last illness that she prayed that God would end his life. She did so while his fellow rabbis and pupils prayed for him to live. When his soul left him and he was relieved of further distress, her actions appear to be the subject of praise. The fourteenth-century authority, Rabbenu Nissim (RaN), takes it as such in his Talmudic commentary (to *N'darim* 40a), and codifies, so to speak, the permission to pray for the death of a person in unmitigated suffering. But a pre-eminent modern authority, R. Eliezer Waldenberg (*Tzitz Eliezer*, V, addendum ch. 5) allows this to everyone *except* to close family members, making the obvious assumption of a conflict of interest. Their own relief from burdens associated with the illness would influence their prayers as much as their concern for the patient. Yale Kamisar was unaware that his conclusion is so halakhic; the argument is undeniable.

Coming back to the Schiavo case, we need to ask what the use of a feeding tube means. Is it medical intervention, that can under some circumstances be undone, or is it an extension of the natural, not medical, need for food and hydration, which it is our duty to continue? A difference of opinion in rabbinic and ethicist groups on this matter has been registered, but R. David Bleich is persuasive of a point of view by his quip—"A feeding tube is no more than Meals on Wheels." The mechanical means by which nutrition and water are administered does not change that need from a basic and natural one to a revocable medical measure. At times the issue is a nasogastric tube, designed for short-term use, which in the longer term could cause aspiration or infection, both potentially fatal, and therefore may and must be removed. This is as opposed to the percutaneous endoscopic gastrostomy tube, the PEG, contemplated for the long run.

The patient's own role begins with the responsibility to preserve one's own life, to seek and accept needed medical attention. The medical profession and the rest of us have a mandate to heal, but the patient has a mandate to be healed. In a previous volume, I set forth how this is not at all in contravention of God's will, as it historically seemed to some people, but in fulfillment of that will, that we be partners in making the world better. We, for example, must perform the *mitzvah* of restoring a lost wallet, or helping the poor, as the Torah ordains, without ascribing the loss of the wallet, or poverty, or social victimization, to God's inexorable will. In the theology of Ethical Monotheism, our mandate is to be active in *Tikkun Olam,* repairing, so to speak, the world's shortcomings. Restoring lost health, Maimonides teaches, is another way of fulfilling the *mitzvah* of *va'hashevoto lo* (Deuteronomy 22:2), of restoring what one has lost, when we have "found" it, in this case, by virtue of medical skills. The *mitzvah* devolves upon the individual, too, to care for and preserve his or her own health.

All this, of course, bears heavily on the related issue of writing a Living Will. If suicide is not an option morally, it follows that one cannot compose a Living Will that calls for termination of life at a set point, say, if and when that life descends to an undesirable level of quality. Choices other than life-or-death may indeed be included, even that between serious medical treatments and non-intervention, but the "do or die" directive is tantamount to literal suicide. Even where the patient is still competent and communicative, his or her non-lethal choices are limited. Part of the mandate to be healed means that treatment, even surgery, that has greater benefit than risk, may not be refused. But where the risk or downside is greater than the benefit, or even if the procedure is merely experimental, the treatment may indeed be refused. This is called *"shev v'al ta'aseh,"* the permission to forgo hazardous surgery, the absence of a duty to invite such intervention.

This calculus also allows us not to treat where it can be argued that treatment could do harm. It's the basis of another clear exception in the matter of a Living Will, namely the Do Not Resuscitate directive. A DNR can be implemented on the consideration that resuscitation will be counter-therapeutic, that the protocol of, say, beating on the chest or other milder procedures can make the patient worse rather than better. Returning to our present case, retaining a feeding tube in the body of a patient, or intubating to begin with, can be undone if there is conviction that the tube may be the cause of infection or other harm. Only such a conviction can give us a moral right to withhold or withdraw such instruments. (A distinction is often made between withholding, where there is more freedom to do so, and withdrawing, where a palpable act of killing seems to take place. But connecting the implement conditionally, namely, doing so with the express intention of withdrawing when no good has come from it, would seem to answer this objection.)

It must be said, however, that the best of Living Wills are not without serious shortcomings. This is due mainly to the fact that there is no way for a person to know now how he or she will feel about a decision that would take effect sometime in the future. It's virtually impossible to know now how we will assess the alternatives available to us when the time comes. It's a truism that people who have imagined what they would choose in a crisis will change their minds drastically when the crisis comes and the options are newly evaluated. Aside from the moral problem that suicide should not be pre-selected, we know from observation that those who have contemplated it earlier feel quite differently when the stark options stare them in the face. (The Schiavo matter suffered not only from allowing a relative to testify as to Terri's expressed wishes, but also by taking an expression of wishes from a different time and set of circumstances to be applied here and now.)

For such reasons, many hospitals are now showing preference for what is more valid and on the mark, namely the appointment of a proxy to make health-care decisions. The proxy is designated in advance as one who knows the patient's personal history and beliefs, and can honestly represent what that patient would want, adjusted to this time and these circumstances. Circumstances, moreover, can pertain not only to the changed state of mind of the patient, but also to the changed state-of-the-art of medicine. A patient at a local hospital, for one example, had executed a Living Will to the effect that he would not allow the use of a respirator if indicated. When he was brought to the hospital, family members in fact appeared the next day to see to it that the directive be obeyed. But the medical staff decided, on penalty of legal action against them, to ignore that directive which seemed so inappropriate to the case at hand. Upon investigation, they found that the patient had written it as a reaction to witnessing others in a long-time state of bedridden confinement, and intent on avoiding that for himself. But in his present situation, the respirator would only be temporary, needed until his brief period of trauma would pass. So the medical staff set aside his request. They would presumably do the same when portable respirators are available widely. These, to be used like pacemakers, would not confine the patient at all to bed or hospital. Such scenarios illustrate the point made above that we cannot be expected to prophesy now how we will feel then, or what unknown circumstances will then be in place.

In fact, *Forced Exit* is the title of a book by Wesley Smith in which he describes the case, among others, of a woman whose Living Will excluded the use of a feeding tube. When it came to that, she recovered her will to live, raised her voice and said, "Please feed me. I'm hungry. I'm thirsty." But she was locked in. "Her earlier expressed sentiments," writes Smith, "ended up costing this non-terminally ill" woman her life.

Awareness of theoretical and practical deficiencies of a Living Will has produced a strong article published in the March-April 2004 issue of the *Hastings Center Report*. Its unambiguous title is "Enough: The Failure of the Living Will." The article is based on several studies of the practicality and effectiveness of the Living Will idea, and has found it severely wanting, for the above and additional reasons. It argues instead for a power-of-attorney arrangement or a surrogate health-care proxy. Indeed, the designated surrogate can address the present questions much better than a pre-written template or document, providing he or she knows the convictions of the patient and can objectively assess the options and their consequences.

Shortcomings in the concept of the Living Will can be somewhat corrected with legislation now being considered by Israel's Knesset, according to recommendations by Dr. Avraham Steinberg and his committee of 58 doctors, scientists, judges, and rabbis. The proposal affirms the prohibition of active euthanasia but allows for ending needless suffering of the terminally ill through the use of upgraded living wills, ethics committees, respirators that turn themselves off with timers, and a computerized data base in which individuals could restate their end-of-life decisions every five years. The "upgraded" Living Will can, at least, include such desired provisions, all subject to the on-the-spot word of the designated proxy.*

---

* Two points of update, as this book approaches publication. The first is is that the above-described Knesset proposal, having passed its final "reading" by an overwhelming majority, is now the law of the land. The second is that the accomplishment in stem-cell research attributed to scientists in South Korea, mentioned on page 74, has been repudiated and withdrawn from the record.

CHAPTER NINE

SUICIDE AND
THE RIGHT TO DIE

Reference to needless suffering, above, turns our attention now to the role of pain. Although we can seek consolation, after the fact, for the presence of pain in our lives, and find that it may serve a purpose like character-building or something of similar value, it must be said that there is no virtue in enduring pain for its own sake or in knowingly allowing it to continue. Even if pain is seen as punishment, or purgation, we are bidden to actively overcome it, and doing so partakes of *pikkuach nefesh*. R. Eliezer Waldenberg (*Tzitz Eliezer* XIII, 87) specifically includes palliation of pain as part of the *mitzvah* to heal. How is this so? Because the therapeutic progress we aim for is impeded by the presence of pain, not to speak of its distracting and dismaying effect on life itself. Still in all, if we are unable to relieve the pain, it cannot be allowed to drive us from life.

I must admit that I have not always felt this way. My own introduction to Jewish medical ethics came at a young age, when I must have been both cynical and brash. It happened when I made a *shivah* condolence visit to a wife who had lost her husband after protracted disease, painful to the end. She narrated that just six months before, his doctor had offered an experimental drug that promised a cure, and wanted her consent to use it for him. She did, but the cure didn't come, and his

final half year was one of unrelieved pain and suffering. I then put the innocent question to her: "If
you knew then what you know now, would you
still have agreed to the use of the new drug?"
"Yes, of course," she said. Here came my imperti-
nence. "But why? All he had from it was six
months of extended pain, and no cure!" She
looked at me with the disdain I deserved, and
said, "I'll tell you, young man. These six months
may have brought him great pain. But that's not
all they brought. In these six months, he lived to
see the marriage of one more child, and to delight
in the arrival of one more grandchild. And I know
without a doubt that the happiness of those mile-
stone experiences penetrated and dissipated his
suffering. They meant far more to his life and
wellbeing than the pain could ever diminish." I
was properly chastised, and turned a corner in my
understanding of the existential issues here.

It goes without saying that imposing pain unnecessarily on others must be avoided. As it happens, a Hebrew form of the word euthanasia was
"coined" in the Talmud long before the Greek
roots were used by Sir Thomas More to form the
compound English term, except that here the
meaning is not killing for reasons of kindness, but
being kind in the necessary act of killing. Even the
convicted criminal, R. Nachman taught (*Sanhedrin*
45a), deserves our compassion. If he must be executed, we give him a narcotic, that he not suffer
pain as he dies. This is in fulfillment of "Love thy
neighbor as thyself" (Leviticus 19:18), which in-

cludes, this Talmudic sage taught, "Choose for him a good death [*mitah yafah*, literally *euthanatos*]."*

Something about enforced pain by the Romans and much about suicide is gleaned from a striking narrative in the Talmud (*Avodah Zarah* 18a). The passage has to do with the martyr-death of R. Chanina ben Teradyon, along with the deaths of several other rabbis who were executed by the Romans for the sin of teaching Torah. Seeing it as a threat to their hegemony, the Romans had forbidden the teaching of Torah on penalty of death, but these rabbis heroically defied the ban. They cited the parable of the fox, who shrewdly seeks to entice fish out of the pond by pointing to some danger in the water. The fish reply that if their life is in danger in the water—their protective element—how much more is it in danger out of the water! The rabbis similarly reasoned that if their lives are threatened when they teach Torah, they are more threatened when they cease to teach it, "for the Torah is our life and the length of our days."

The Romans paid no attention to this homily

---

* This consideration could be added to the others that militate against the claim that "the Jews killed Jesus." Not only was the *Sanhedrin* not allowed to meet at night, nor was it allowed to meet on a holiday such as Passover, but certainly it was not permitted to (violate "love thy neighbor" and) give over an accused person to a crucifixion or to a painful death. The agony of the Passion as celebrated by its producer in a recent movie is ethically and literally worlds removed from the universe of Jewish practice.

and proceeded to execute the offending rabbis, but never without the harshest of added torture. In the case of R. Chanina ben Teradyon, he was placed in the fire for execution, but first his chest was covered with woolen sponges drenched in water. This would delay his death while the flames burned and thus prolong his agony. His disciples pleaded with him to overcome this evil device by opening his mouth wide so that he might be asphyxiated by the smoke, die more quickly, and be spared a few minutes of pain. He refused, says the narrative, on the grounds that such would constitute suicide. "Only He Who gave life can take it away. I may not do so myself," he replied to his disciples in this incredible conversation.

"Well then," the executioner intervened, offering an alternative. "Let me remove these moistened sponges around your heart" that the painful dying not be prolonged. That, R. Chanina indicated, is permissible. The first suggestion was an act of suicide, of hastening death by one's own actions. That he would not do. The second was a case of removing an impediment, artificially supplied, which delayed the expected process of dying. That would be the allowable removal of a hindrance to "natural" death. The executioner did so, and R. Chanina's agony ended. When the executioner himself died, the Talmud declares, he "went straight to heaven" for this act of exquisite mercy—implying, of course, that the act was not only permissible but praiseworthy. We are even told that the eminent R. Judah Ha-Nasi spoke enviously of him. Some of us, he said, strive throughout our lifetimes to earn a share in the World to Come, but some earn their place there in "a single moment" of great righteousness!

The narrative found its way into the codes of *halakhah*, where the implicit teachings were made explicit. To hasten death is not permitted. To "remove hindrances" to the "soul's departure" is permitted and even mandated. While physicians, to state the matter in contemporary terms, may not disconnect life-support systems where that shortens life, they may do so to shorten the death process. Since death is a process rather than an event, and since "we begin dying the moment we are born," and, more to the point, it's difficult to tell the difference between prolonging life and prolonging death, the principle is often a moral one more than a practical one.

Compassion in the relief of pain is indeed the ethical imperative. The Hastings Institute, a pioneer agency for the study of medical ethics, now makes the point that advances in pain-relief technology—while greater progress remains to be made—have radically reduced the number of instances in which pain might justify recourse to euthanasia. The Institute was happy to hear that, from the standpoint of *halakhah*, pain relief is essential, but administering it in order to accelerate death is not allowed. That is, while hastening death remains forbidden—as either an active or passive intentional act—rabbinic authorities are unanimous in permitting the use of analgesics for the purpose of relieving pain. This is so, even if doing so knowingly shortens life, because the intent is mercy for life, not for killing. Intent makes all the difference.

To clarify further, we are bidden by the Talmudic teaching to stand in the tradition of our forefather Abraham, to be *"rachamanim, bayyshanim, gom'lei chasadim*—merciful, reverent, and doers of deeds of kindness." So, the very phrase, "mercy killing," needs to be parsed; the two words need to be disjoined. Mercy, mercy, in all things, at all times, except where it involves the evil of intentional killing. That's a line that mercy cannot cross. Interesting is the commentary on the Biblical verse addressed to Noah's descendants who were to rebuild the world, after the Flood. They were admonished against "the spilling of the blood of mankind, the spilling of the blood of one's brother." The added phrase, says the commentary, is to forbid murder even for "brotherly" reasons, for reasons of brotherly compassion.

In a recent exchange in the Op-Ed pages of the New York Times, Dr. Thomas A. Preston, a cardiologist, called into question the supposed difference between so-called physician-assisted suicide on the one hand and administration of morphine to relieve pain, on the other. The latter, he claimed, leads just as certainly to shortening one's life. To which Dr. Kenneth Prager responded emphatically—there's all the difference in the world between the two. He referred to his own experience in the practice of pulmonology over many decades, in which he would calibrate the dosage of morphine as needed to relieve the pain. If death sometimes nonetheless followed as a result thereof, there had been no intent to kill, only an intent to palliate pain. Intent is everything; again, it is where killing is morally distinct from murdering. True, the victim is "just as dead" whether the cause was an act of murder or an act of unintentional killing, but the perpetrator avoids killing himself spiritually by keeping far from an act of willful murder.

My Catholic colleagues point out that we are more liberal than they on abortion, they more liberal than we on euthanasia. This may or may not be so, but I am proud of the salutation *"l'chayyim,"* expressing this Jewish reverence for life, and confidently urge it on those who must face difficult decisions. Its point, as offered in Chapter 1, is a profounder sanctification of life. It issues from an abhorrence of murder, as well as awesome reverence for the image of God within us. Nonetheless, this foundational principle is not absolute; it leaves room for necessary, if limited, martyrdom. Remarkably, murder of the innocent is a cardinal sin, one of the three the avoidance of which requires martyrdom instead. I may set aside the entire Torah to save a life (*ya'avor v'al yehareg*) but, rather than commit murder of an innocent life, I must rather martyr myself to avoid that (*yehareg v'al ya'avor*). This means, at least in theory, that I must surrender my life to protect the principle of not taking life! (And even this extreme of "surrender of one's life" is still above "taking one's life.") So it's not the number of lives forfeited, but the preservation of the principle not to take an innocent life. In the face of widespread human violence, and yes, even in view of catastrophic natural disasters, all of which seem to cheapen life, we are bidden with our actions to hold it sacred and inviolate.

Aside from the high moral ground in holding life inviolate as a principle, there are eminently practical grounds for resisting the surrender thereof in, for example, suicide or assisted suicide. A right to die, legislatively enacted, would not be a favor to us. Under such a law, we would be forced to consider choosing that right. As an example, the following scenario could become routine: A son says to his father, "Dad, Uncle Ted didn't put us through this ordeal when he was about to die. Why don't you be a good dad and do what he did?" An active termination of life could follow, by his signaling the physician to that effect. Or, even an inactive one: The father unclenches his fists, gives up the fight and the will to live, and the right to live. Here, too, the children have enabled a premature death. In all such situations, how do we keep the right to die from becoming the duty to die? Once the choice is given to us, how do we resist the pressure to go ahead and make that choice? Or, escape the guilt for not doing so?

Prof. Leon Kass offers a related point in his book, *Toward a More Natural Science*: "For, the choice for death is not one option among many, but an option to end all options. Socially, there will be great pressure on the aged and the vulnerable to exercise this option." Writing recently in *Commentary* magazine, he argued further that once there looms the legal alternative of euthanasia, it will plague every decision made by any seriously-ill elderly person—not to speak of their more powerful caretakers—even without the subtle hints and pressures applied to them by others.

There is, in fact, much to be learned from the public discussion of euthanasia. The saddest part of the first Kevorkian case is the suicide note of Janet Adkins, mentioned above, which was printed on the front page of The New York Times. She wrote that the threat of worsening Alzheimer's disease made her fear becoming a burden to her family. The threat, that is. She therefore asked that her life be snuffed out long before she would enter the dependent stage. But that very idea is an ominous one. Anyone's fear of becoming a burden is manifestly undeserved, and should not be encouraged; it should not be determinative in our attitude to life and death. People with severe or with lesser afflictions, who have "paid their dues," and presumably have given life and help to others, deserve our nurture and care, without being made to feel they are a burden. That would be an indictment of the rest of us. The *mitzvah* of *bikkur cholim*, of visiting the sick, fulfills many vital purposes. Among them is the assurance it gives to proud people, who have now been rendered dependent, that they share our right to life and are entitled to our return of respectful caring.

Having said all of the above, it must be noted that there is a category in Jewish law of *patur aval asur*, meaning a transgression which is unpunishable but nonetheless forbidden. Its obverse is *asur aval patur*, something that is forbidden but nonetheless unpunishable. This is how Jewish law ultimately deals with the deed of suicide. As a deterrent, we are told that the sin of suicide calls for the punitive denial to the person of funeral obsequies, such as eulogies and even *shivah* observance. After the fact, however, the perpetrator is judged to have been under such psychological pressure, so depressively distraught, that he was not in command of his actions. The deed is therefore forgiven, and the funeral and post-funeral honors are to be granted.

Yes, the act of suicide could have been a conscious and knowing one, a philosophic rejection of values of right and wrong. But, especially if the deed could not be rationally controlled, the person committed an act that remains forbidden but he must be forgiven. Consider the unexpected phrase for suicide—it is *m'abbed atzmo la-da'at* "to do away with oneself consciously," with that last word adding the factor of full awareness. For those cases of serious deterioration of quality of life, however, or in the presence of intractable pain, the theoretical categorization of suicide remains *asur* as a policy, but when it is genuinely unavoidable or uncontrollable, then he or she is *patur* of wrongdoing; the deed cannot be held against the hapless person. For one's "share in the

World to Come," the hope is that divine judgment will be as compassionate as that of the earthly court.

Indeed, there are undeniably situations where death could be called preferable to continued life in distress. The *midrash* alludes to this idea by means of a similar-in-sound, but not similar-in-meaning, pair of words. The text in Genesis 1:31 says "and God saw all that He had made, and behold it was very good," where the concluding Hebrew phrase is *"tov m'od."* The *midrash* allows one to read it as *"tov mot,"* meaning that "death is good." A philosophic perspective, but not a sentiment to act upon. As has been said, suicide provides a permanent solution to a temporary problem. A town in New Jersey recently reported the episode of a suicide pact shared by four teenagers. At the pre-arranged cue, they all honored the pact and took their own lives. Whatever it could have been that led them, or other university students recently in the news, to this deed was certainly something of a temporary, passing nature. But their lost lives are forever irretrievable. In the face of such tragedy, we may marshal greater sympathy for the young who make this mistake. But the principle of no chance to reconsider is the same for them as for older or more compromised lives.

For, even if death is indeed seen to be good, we are not allowed to bring it about in ourselves, just as we are not allowed to bring it about in others. Homicide does not become permissible just because we deem someone unworthy of living, and suicide is not that different. Again, details of the *halakhah* make it clear: Having come to the conclusion that the life of a loved one is unbearable, may one pray to God that He bring the life to an end? Surprisingly, the answer is yes, as we saw in the previous chapter. When death does come, may we offer thanks to God for that outcome? The answer is again yes. We may pray for the relief that death brings; we may thank God when that relief comes. What we may not do is bring about death actively; we cannot do it *b'yadayim*, with our own hands.

The famous example of Masada might come to mind in objection to the above. The defenders of the fortress Masada, the last outpost in the Jewish war with Rome, are said to have chosen to take their own lives rather than submit to the depredations of the Romans. But scholars, such as Trude Weiss-Rosmarin and others, deny this ever happened. They remind us that the lone source available to us for the whole narrative was that of the historian Josephus, who needed to acquit himself for having fled the scene. Nonetheless, Masada has become a symbol of fearless resistance and remained so into modern times. But it must be noted that the event and its assessment evoked no reflection at all in halakhic literature.

The negative attitude to suicide is actually the other side of the coin of our vaunted principle of *pikkuach nefesh*. The mandate of this principle is to do almost everything to save life—including to protect it from our own aggression.

CHAPTER TEN

SOME CONCLUDING THOUGHTS

The practical guidance of *halakhah* on the questions addressed here is consistent, not haphazard or contradictory. Jewish law and morality are rather predictable in their defining positions, once the factors involved are sifted and analyzed. What emerges is a steadfast commitment to maintaining life, even when that clashes with the moment's ritual obligations, and to faithfully guard existing life while pursuing other legitimate and recommended deeds

The striking message is that virtually all the *mitzvot* or otherwise good pursuits, or restrictions, must be set aside if danger to life or health presents itself. We are being taught that *pikkuach nefesh* comes first and displaces all else. Outside of the rare cases where martyrdom is allowed, the *mitzvah* of safeguarding our health or the health of those around us comes ahead of any other consideration. The Sabbath, Holidays, Yom Kippur, dietary laws, ritual requirements of all kinds, stand aside in the presence of the need to avert a threat to life. Physical danger and substantive mental danger, or therapeutic need, must be addressed before ritual demands can resume. Since the average person is not an expert in diagnosis, even what is only possibly dangerous must be removed. The *halakhah* generally makes liberal allowance, so that we err on the side of safety.

But if Torah laws must be set aside to save life, it surely does not follow that they may be set aside to take life. In the chapter on abortion and stem cell research, it was made clear that preserving the existing life of the mother takes precedence over the potential life of the fetus. That is to say, natalism and procreation are great values, but they are not to be encouraged if they threaten existing life. *Chatam Sofer* was quoted, in response to a question, that, as much as these values are desirable even for one to whom pregnancy is life-threatening, "no woman is required to build the world by destroying herself." In difficult historical times for Jewish women, when poverty or oppression made childbirth a real challenge, they rose to the challenge and met it heroically. But when life or health was threatened, they were bidden to yield to the principle of *pikkuach nefesh* to protect their own existing life. Hence, while casual abortion gets no sanction, the *halakhah* of mandated abortion demonstrates that the existing life of the mother cannot be sacrificed to the misplaced notion of abortion as murder.

This helps us understand, even if we don't at all subscribe to it, the position of those such as President George W. Bush who oppose research on embryonic stem cells. From our standpoint it is clear that human life begins much later in the gestational process, and the pre-implantational stage does not yet bring the embryo from potential to actual human life. But for those who find humanness to begin earlier, their position reflects their conviction that even the promise of life-saving therapeutic help should not come at the expense of life now. Similarly, although the analogy is a daring one, the chapter here on determination of death is slanted towards those rabbinic authorities who accept brain death in order to permit the life-saving effort of heart transplantation. But respect is due as well to those who fear that existing life yet lingers in the heart donor, and that *pikkuach nefesh* for the donee cannot justify the action, even with the best motives in the world.

Looking to another set of issues, respect for the body of the deceased, which until just recently housed the soul and continues to be associated with a specific personality, is also a sacred value. It can be overruled in the name of saving a life through the help that autopsy yields or through the health that a transplant provides. But we are taught to ensure that there be a close and necessary connection between the medical procedure and the benefit, so that *k'vod ha-met* not be compromised unless it brings *pikkuach nefesh*. In still another chapter, we saw that even the objection to onanistic contraceptive means could be addressed, if that were the only way to safeguard the health of the wife and, at the same time, encourage marital relations rather than abstinence.

Overall, the awe and trepidation that keeps us from shortening an existing life because of medical futility or diminished quality asserts itself in the name of the sanctity of life. We treasure the quality of *rachamanut*; mercy is a primary quality to have and to cultivate, but it has to stop short at the doorstep of killing. The mercy we advocate is the kind that allows for non-intervention at strategic times, expressed during lucid consultations or in Living Will directives, in exclusion of active euthanasia and despairing suicide. It can even be said that true mercy inheres in our opposition to legalized euthanasia or physician-assisted suicide. For, once these are legally available, the right to die becomes the duty to die, and the patient has to explain why that path was not chosen; he or she has to resist the pressure or bear the guilt.

We need to address pain and suffering by increased pain-management research and attention, as well as by adopting the attitude suggested here that life is precious in spite of pain. And, the administering of adequate morphine to alleviate pain is a *mitzvah*, while to do so to end a life is a sin. Even if the outcome is inevitable, the intent is what's determinative. Intent is everything, even though the patient is "just as dead." If we knowingly bring about a person's death, we kill ourselves spiritually by having transgressed the boundary between killing and murdering.

A hard-to-absorb passage in *Talmud Yerushalmi* (*T'rumot* 8:12) was not included in the presentation of the chapters above. It teaches that if a contingent of Jews is "besieged by heathens who declare 'Give us one of your company and we shall kill him; if not, we will kill all of you,' let them all be killed, but let them not deliver [to the enemy] a single Jewish soul." The passage goes on to imply that if the captors had asked for one who they say has a warrant against him (as with Sheba the son of Bichri in II Samuel 20:22), that's different. Looking at the first part, we wonder why several lives should be forfeit where we can escape by losing just one? The answer is that the principle of not killing the innocent, or not cooperating in such killing, is so important that life itself must be surrendered. It is not the number of lives that makes the difference, but honoring the principle that murder should be unthinkable. As in the martyrdom expected for resisting the order to murder the innocent (*yehareg v'al ya'avor*), it's not the loss of life but the violence against the moral principle that needs to be prevented.

All this supports the doctrine that life is sacred, and this manifesto should even help to bolster self-esteem. In the face of threats to life and actions that demean it, we stress its sanctity and uniqueness, its preciousness and inalienability, because we are creatures in the image of God. In the face of our own humility and relative insignificance, we see life as a gift for us to cherish and hold high. We have the duty to take good care of ourselves and build good health and preserve life, and to be its guardians in both sickness and health. The hierarchy of values we have inherited as our tradition makes it imperative that we raise these goals above even spiritual ones, because we know what Maimonides has taught: It is a duty to tend the material body so that it can pursue the spiritual goals.

The end of Chapter Three cited Maimonides on a different point. We were intrigued and impressed by what he wrote in characterizing the Torah's laws of *pikkuach nefesh*, of setting aside restrictions for the possibility of saving life or health. He wrote that this shows that the Torah's teachings are not *n'kamah*, "vengeance" or "vindictiveness," against the world, but the opposite. Actually, they demonstrate that the motif of *"va-chai bahem,* one... shall live by them" in Leviticus is about bringing mercy and kindness and wholeness to the world. In our quest for an answer to what prompted Maimonides to include in his legal code a thought so theological or even polemical, we find scholars who suggest that certain heretical sects in his time preached otherwise. Perhaps so. But the uplifting idea stands on its own. Our Torah is a Tree of Life that bids us exalt and preserve life, not undermine nor underrate it.

We are sorely tempted to abandon our reverence for life in the face of mass killings by murderous oppressors or at the experience of natural disasters in their various forms. Implied in the above Talmudic paradigm is the teaching that, as much as human life is vulnerable in these ways, we will not betray the mandate to cherish and value a single life. Even for a momentary span or an ebbing phase of life we will afford the same adequate treatment and adequate appreciation. The teaching extends as well to the conviction that we are fully entitled to the care and attention of others without being seen as a burden.

As of the moment of this conclusory writing, Prof. Leon Kass, in stepping down from the chairmanship of the President's Council on Bioethics, summarized the moral harvest of the Council's deliberations. In a rebuke to what it decries as growing individualism, the document holds high the worth of relationships and of mutual neediness and dependence. It even touches upon the writing of Living Wills and finds them to be a rejection of wholesome dependence and reciprocal assistance, reminding us that "giving care always requires more in terms of resources, character, support and judgment than any legal instrument can possibly provide." Unchanging in the face of evolving instruments and attitudes is the sacred principle that, to each other, we are not a burden, not expendable, not a mere number, but fellow human beings with a spark of the Divine.

L'chayyim!

ADDENDUM

As this volume is being prepared, much earlier than expected, for its second printing, I take the opportunity to add here some points of further illustration of its major themes.

The extraordinary force of the *pikkuach nefesh* principle is best seen in the halakhic ruling for a suffering patient for whose demise we are in fact permitted to pray (see page 104), such release being the only way to end the pain. The Sabbath may nonetheless be violated for this patient — "even several times" — on the off-chance that that may still avail, says R. Shlomoh Zalman Auerbach (*Minchat Shlomoh* Vol. 1, 91:24). He makes this paradoxical judgment after once again affirming eloquently life's infinite value.

In discussing the matter of a Living Will and its usual attestation that its writer wants treatment to cease if the disease progresses to a certain point, and in connection with our observation that one's wishes are seldom the same when arriving at that eventuality, it is highly interesting to read what is said in connection with Peter Singer of Princeton University. In a book called *Do As I Say (Not As I Do)*, the author Peter Schweitzer offers what he calls "Profiles in Liberal Hypocrisy." As opposed to the other examples in his book, the kind of "hypocrisy" that he welcomes is the following: Singer is known for advocating infanticide and euthanasia for the handicapped or disabled; "people with a whole host of ailments, including Alzheimer's... should have their lives ended prematurely." Then Schweitzer learned that Singer's own mother has Alzheimer's, but then, "far from embracing his own moral ethic, Singer hired a group of health care workers to look after her."

The heated dispute about abortion policy continues unabated. This book sets forth the Jewish legal-moral position as "pro-life," which, before that became a slogan, meant that existing life, i.e. the mother's, must be preserved when in contest with that of potential life, i.e. the fetus. But the mother's life also mans the mother's health, and the rabbis ruled for abortion in the case of her physical and serious mental health. We cited the words of *Chatam Sofer* to the effect that "No woman should be asked to build the world (in becoming pregnant) by destroying herself." In current debates, the issue of abortion for rape victims has come to the fore, and opponents say that if abortion is murder, there is no remedy for such victims. In this regard another rabbinic statement that sounds like a "feminist manifesto" should be introduced: Rabbi Yerucham Perilman, the *"Gadol of Minsk,"* wrote (Responsa *Or Gadol*, No. 31) that whereas a woman is a vehicle of reproduction, like mother earth (*karka olam*), she obviously differs in that she is human, and should not be asked to nurture seed implanted in her against her will.

GLOSSARY

asur	forbidden
bar kayyama	a viable infant
Bavli	Babylonian Talmud
bikkur cholim	visiting the sick
Binyan Tziyyon	Responsa of R. Jacob Ettlinger
b'rit	circumcision
b'yadayyim	with [your own] hands
chamira sakkanta me-issura	danger to life is graver than ritual infraction
chareidim	"fervently Orthodox"
Chatam Sofer	"Chiddushei Torat Mosheh," R. Moses Sofer (d. 1839)
chayyei sha'ah	momentary life

choleh l'faneinu	a patient before us
Even HaEzer	section of the Code of Jewish Law
Gaon	a rabbi of the post-Talmudic Geonic period; or, here, a rare scholar
goses	moribund
halakhah	Jewish law (adjective form: halakhic)
halanat ha-met	delaying burial
ha-n'shamah she-b'mochi	the soul in my brain
Haskalah	The Enlightenment movement
Hatzalah	Rescue service
ha-zariz	the diligent one
Iggerot Mosheh	Responsa of R. Mosheh Feinstein
kavvanah	intention-focusing
kibbud em	honor due to mother
K'nesset	Israel's law-making body
k'vod ha-met	respect for the dead
l'chayyim	to life

lo taharog	thou shalt not kill
lo tirtzach	thou shalt not murder
m'abbed atzmo la-da'at	takes one's own life
midrash	rabbinic exegesis not necessarily in the Talmud
Minchat Chinnukh	Commentary to Sefer HaChinnukh
Mishnah	foundational statement of Jewish law
(adjective form: Mishnaic)	which, with G'mara, "the learning," constitutes the Talmud
Minchat Shlomoh	Responsa of R. Shlomoh Zalman Auerbach
mishum eivah	to prevent enmity
mitah yafah	a good death
mitzvah (plural: mitzvot)	a commandment, or a good deed
mohel	b'rit practitioner
mot yamut	he shall surely die
nefesh	a soul / a person

nivvul ha-met	desecration of the dead
n'kamah	vindictiveness
Orach Chayyim	a section of the Code of Jewish Law
patur	exempt
pikkuach nefesh	saving life or health
p'ru ur'vu	be fruitful and multiply
p'sik reisheih v'lo yamut	"if you cut off its head will it not die?"
rachamanut	mercy
Rambam	R. Moses Maimonides (d. 1204)
Ramban	R. Moses Nachmanides (d. 1268)
RaN	R. Nissim Girondi (d. 1380)
Rashi	R. Shlomoh Yitzchaki (d. 1105)
rodef	a pursuer
safek pikkuach nefesh	possible saving of life or health
she-hecheyanu	He hath kept us in life
sh'loshah she-ach'lu	"three who ate"
Shulchan Arukh	The Code of Jewish Law

shivah	the week of mourning
Talmud	Mishnah plus G'mara. The many volumes of legal and extralegal interpretation and application of Torah by the rabbis over several centuries. (See "Bavli" and "Yerushalmi").
t'chiyyat ha-metim	resurrection of the dead
t'fillin	"phylacteries"
teruf da'at	mental instability
Tosafot	critical commentary to Talmud
Tzitz Eliezer	Responsa of R. Eliezer Waldenberg
va-chai ba-hem	"and live by them"
viddui	confessional
ya'avor v'al yehareg	let him transgress and not be martyred
yehareg v'al ya'avor	let him be martyred and not transgress
Yerushalmi	Palestinian Talmud
yichus	lineage
Yom Tov	religious holiday

Yoreh Deah	section of the Code of Jewish Law
z'nav ha-l'taah	the lizard's tail
zochreinu l'chayyim	remember us to life

SUBJECT INDEX

NAME INDEX

ABOUT THE AUTHOR

Rabbi David M. Feldman is Dean of the Jewish Institute of Bioethics. He is the author of *Birth Control in Jewish Law: Marital Relations, Contraception and Abortion, As Set Forth in the Classic Texts of Jewish Law*, published by New York University Press in 1968. It then appeared in several paperback editions under the title *Marital Relations*, etc., and has now been republished in augmented form, updating its material on new fertility questions and returning to its original title plus "Third Edition — With Epilogue 1995". He is also the author of *The Jewish Family Relationship* and *Health and Medicine in the Jewish Tradition*, the latter commissioned by the Lutheran Institute of Human Ecology and published by Crossroad. He is the Editor of the *Compendium on Medical Ethics* and has written several articles for the *Encyclopedia Judaica* and for both the original 1978 edition of the *Encyclopedia of Bioethics* and for its revised 1995 edition.

Dr. Feldman pursued graduate studies at Columbia and at the University of Illinois, and holds degrees from Yeshiva University and the Jewish Theological Seminary, as well as *semikhah* from Rav Natalovitch. Having served as chaplain in the U.S. Air Force and then for many years as Rabbi of the Bay Ridge Jewish Center in Brooklyn, he is now Rabbi Emeritus of the Jewish Center of Teaneck, New Jersey. He was recently granted the "Rabbi of the Year" Award by the New York Board of Rabbis.

Rabbi Feldman has served as Chairman of the Committee on Medical Ethics of UJA-Federation and as Chairman of its Committee on Marriage and the Family. A long-standing member of the Law Committee of the Rabbinical Assembly, he served on the faculty of the School for Chaplains of the New York Board of Rabbis and as Visiting Associate Professor at the Jewish Theological Seminary. He is a Founding Fellow of the Hastings Institute of Society, Ethics, and the Life Sciences and a member of the Editorial Advisory of the Encyclopedia of Bioethics, sponsored by the Kennedy Institute. He also serves on the Bio-Medical Ethics Committee of Hackensack University Medical Center and on the Board of Trustees of the New York Society for the Deaf.

Dr. Feldman has lectured widely before synagogue, university, and medical groups. He gave testimony in Albany and Washington on abortion and population issues. He was invited to Rome to address a Vatican-sponsored conference on the subject of his first book and delivered a series of lectures on Jewish law at the Law School of the Hebrew University in Jerusalem.